The world needs warriors

Being a Weightloss Warrior is about learning how to react, controlling your reaction to food choices, as well as to emotional turmoil, stress and activity. Today more than ever we are constantly assailed by toxic food, toxic people and toxic environments.

Weightloss warriors empower themselves through quality choices and don't guilt themselves into binge exercising or extreme fasting. A weightloss warrior—as opposed to a fitness soldier—understands the personal journey they are on towards a healthy body and mind. A warrior makes conscious choices—understanding how each will affect their metabolism, their hormones and their happiness. They don't beat themselves up over stray kilos or unrealistic goals and they never exercise out of guilt or shame themselves into deprivation. And they certainly don't mindlessly follow a fad diet, someone else's gruelling training regime, or allow others to dictate a course of action without listening to their own body!

I live by the ancient philosophy of 'hard training, easy combat'. Like challenging yourself in the dojang: genuinely taking on your emotional enemies while training means the mind is prepared for the challenge of combat, and everything in life becomes easier. The battle is over before it's begun. And you are the winner!

But the only one who can unleash this awesome inner warrior is you (with a little of my help, of course!). No one is born a warrior; instead, you become one through small private victories that eventually lead to overcoming great challenges.

NinjaMove
GO ELEMENTAL

Earth: discover the power of eating food 'naked'—go natural and get grounded. You eat pure energy when you consume quality, vital, raw ingredients.

Fire: engage your metabolism, develop your lean muscle mass, balance your heat and restore your hormones. Metabolic harmony recharges and redirects our energy, training the inside first and then the outside.

Wind: experience the pleasure of movement. Exercise equals happiness, which equates to freedom. Feel truly powerful.

Water: channel the power of positive thinking and enjoy the benefits of complete hydration. Your thoughts are flexible, changeable, mutable—like water—and shape who you are today.

WARRIOR WEAPONS

Health is your armour: Physical and mental health, as well as emotional fitness, will protect the warrior on their weightloss journey.

Your tribe is your support network: The warrior's greatest asset is their tribe—your family and friends. You must support them in order to be supported by them. A healthy YOU is a healthy family; a healthy community means healthier choices for the healthiest planet.

Passion is your weapon: Find your passion; then live for it. Your passion should be your compass that navigates your journey through life. It is your purpose and will protect you against all enemies, all defeats and all challenges.

Why taekwondo

The philosophy of taekwondo is about becoming one with the universe: living in harmony with your surroundings and yourself. If you're not at peace with your environment or emotions then you shield yourself from your inner and outer worlds. You stop listening to your body and repress your feelings. The Yin and Yang of taekwondo symbolise universal harmony and balance, in which the passive and active, the feminine and the masculine, form one whole. It's when this balance falls out of whack that problems arise—like putting on weight.

Chi is the vital energy force inherent in all things. According to traditional Chinese medicine, a balance of negative and positive chi circulates in the body and is essential for health and happiness. To be a weightloss warrior we must find our inner chi by tuning in to our body. Being overweight isn't just about food: it's also about feelings. Food has become an antidepressant, or an anaesthetic. An addiction, even. When you feel pain, discomfort, or just plain old hunger you can respond appropriately, but if you repress your feelings you can't control your responses to them. Inner awareness is the core of lasting weight loss and controlling your energy flow. You lose energy because of nutritionally void foods, frustrating relationships or aggravating environments. Positive chi attracts positive chi. Inner mantras of power, presence and light radiate our chi outwards to others. A healthy body is a beautiful body; when you feel great you look sensational.

The art of taekwondo begins with the individual and works to develop the character and positive moral and ethical traits of each practitioner upon this solid foundation. The individual warrior can then pass onto others, through teachings and personal actions, the principles they've learned through their training. Individuals unite and become a family; families bind together and form a community; communities merge and develop into nations; and nations become healthier and more harmonious as a result. It's the physical, mental and spiritual effort that you invest in your training that makes this possible and worthwhile.

WARRIOR CODE

Respect: love your body and your body will love you back.

Passion: follow your passion; let it be your compass in life.

Control: take control of who you are and so control who you will become.

Confidence: warriors are not forged in battle; they are forged in the mind. Believe yourself to be a warrior: powerful in body, centred in spirit and mentally strong.

Commitment: commit to constant and never-ending improvement.

Discipline: train your mind and your mind will train your body.

Habit: create winning habits by making empowered, healthy choices.

Focus: focus on fitness with meaning, not just fat loss (knowing that focus precedes success).

Voice: understand that your greatest enemy lies within. Conquer it by speaking to yourself with love, respect and honour.

Value: value yourself and, in doing so, add value to your tribe.

The metamorphosis of the individual is a process of steps. The progression of belts is symbolic of mental and physical growth, five levels of mastery that practitioners don't simply pass through but add to: from the introductory white belt to yellow's skill, blue's commitment, red's passion and, finally, the black belt's statement of self-mastery and adherence to the Warrior Code.

If you are struggling with your weight, you may have been fighting with yourself for years. Fighting temptation, fighting low self-esteem, fighting bad habits, fighting addictions and fighting eroding confidence. That's exhausting. The fight is not with yourself, but *for* yourself. It's not against fat, it's *for* fitness.

Are you ready to unleash your inner warrior? It's only when you truly love your body, and attach the deepest meaning to your weight loss, that your body will love you back with more energy, more beauty, more years of life, and yes—less fat!

GET YA NINJA ON!

More about me

My family—living their lives in white taekwondo uniforms and driving around in vans emblazoned with 'Hall's Taekwondo'— is fuelled by passion and absolutely focused on fitness with meaning. My parents have helped raise an army of empowered ninjas, giving every student at their schools the gift of self-confidence and resilience. As a little girl, my day started with before-breakfast breathing exercises on the nature strip to expel the stale night air before joining the entire school in 'Fitness for Fun' sessions before assembly run by—yup, you guessed it—my parents!

Other winning habits passed on include 'move fast to stay young' (we didn't walk through department stores, we ran), Hulk juice, (a concoction of spirulina and green vegies blended in water to 'cleanse out the clog'), seizing any opportunity to stretch (waiting in lines at the bank or at the supermarket checkout), carrying fresh fruit into the cinemas (in protest of the candy bar), a ban on 'slow food' (which I now know everyone else calls fast food, because of how you get it and not what it does to you) and membership to what my parents called the Gym of Life … all of which I'm about to pass on to you.

Because it's never too late to grow up ninja!

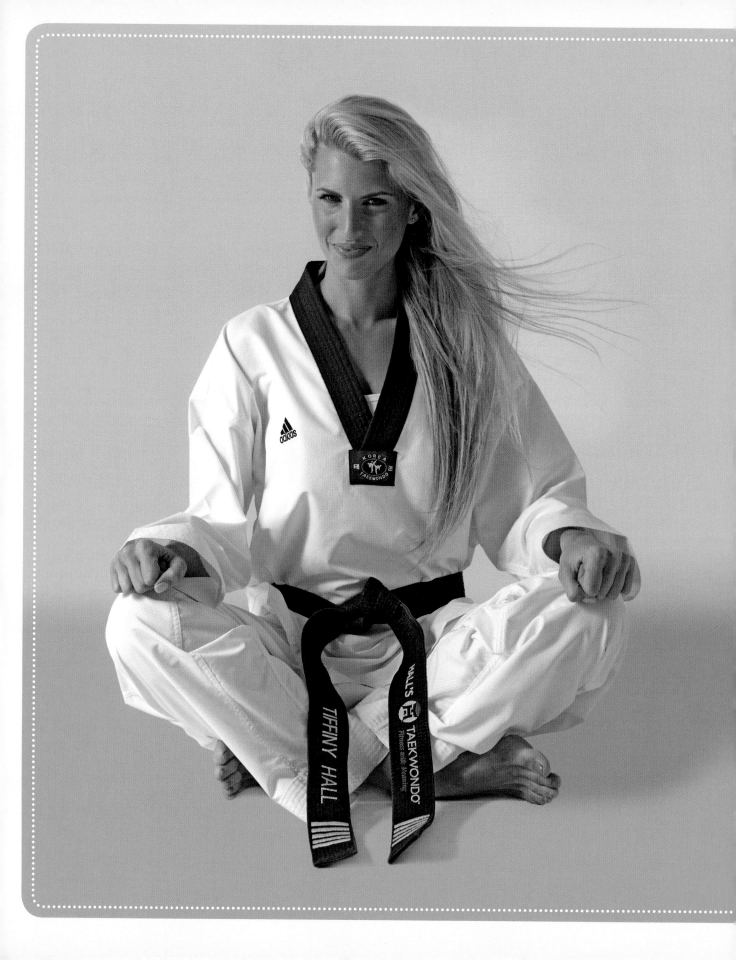

White belt: Warrior mindset

'WHEN YOU ARE THE BEST YOU CAN BE EVERYTHING AROUND YOU GROWS RICHER. YOUR RELATIONSHIPS IMPROVE, YOUR CONFIDENCE SOARS AND OPPORTUNITIES IN LIFE UNFOLD'

Preparing for battle

My approach to weight loss and improved health is as much psychological as it is physical. I believe thoughts transform your body. A fighting-fit body begins with a supple, flexible mind. When you make over your mind you will transform your body and change your life. So, weightloss warriors, where do we start?

Every warrior needs a weapon. You can't fight, let alone win, any battles unarmed. Without the power of self-renewal the body becomes weak, the mind mechanical, the emotions raw, the spirit insensitive and the person selfish. One of the warrior's greatest weapons is an approach I call Sharpening the Sword. When you balance your health habits you equip yourself with the razor-sharp weapon of self-renewal, which creates growth and produces change, giving you the power you need to stick to the warrior code. This in turn strengthens your resolve to progress from the beginner's white belt through to the black belt of self-mastery.

Remember, the battle and the enemy are both within.

Choose your teachers

If I want to be the best at something, or if I want to learn something new, I seek out the warrior masters who came before me. In career, life, health and personal excellence, there's no harm in asking successful people to share their strategies, journeys or secrets with you. Do what they did. Read what they read, or what they've written. Teach yourself to think the way they think.

Emulate success to be successful. Be the master mime of a mastermind! In things you fear, seek out others who have become fearless. Unsuccessful people are unsure; successful people are successful because they have certainty.

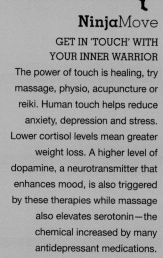

NinjaMove

GET IN 'TOUCH' WITH YOUR INNER WARRIOR

The power of touch is healing, try massage, physio, acupuncture or reiki. Human touch helps reduce anxiety, depression and stress. Lower cortisol levels mean greater weight loss. A higher level of dopamine, a neurotransmitter that enhances mood, is also triggered by these therapies while massage also elevates serotonin—the chemical increased by many antidepressant medications.

WARRIOR SPIRIT

There's no such thing as failure—only finding a new direction.

Halfway through an operation, surgery can look like murder. In the middle of any journey it can seem like the path is lost—end results are rarely obvious early on. But on the road to weight loss there really is no failure: if you are achieving the result you want, you know you are on track; if you aren't, you have learnt how things don't work for you and know you have to change direction. The journey lasts your whole life long. Warriors never surrender or give up—they just get tougher. So be flexible in your approach and persistent in your actions. No one is born a warrior, but we can become one via a slow process of constant negotiation with our inner selves and self-defeating ways.

Renew your honour

Values lie at the core of everything you are and do. Your values are the unifying principles and core beliefs of your personality and directly determine your character. Your values are the points on the compass that will guide you on your warrior path. Life change and body transformation begin with clarifying your true values, and then committing yourself to live according to them. When you value and improve yourself you add value to your tribe—if you're a parent it's not selfish to take time out to unleash your inner warrior: when you are happy and healthy and mentally and physically powerful, then your kids will become so too.

But to achieve your goal it must fit with your beliefs. If you want to lose weight because you believe it's important to be healthy, and you value health as beauty, then it will be easy to master your meals and move your body. But if you only want to lose weight to be a specific dress size for someone's wedding, then the fear of failing and the feeling of worthlessness that comes with that are incongruent with long-term weight loss. Vanity, fear and self-loathing lead to emotional weight-gain and *never* lasting fat loss. Fear is a powerful force, but not one that spurs you towards greatness or lightness.

We can all get quite bitter and miserable when we're weighed down by baggage—some of which we've taken on, and some of which we may have been given. Free yourself up to focus on the fun! The world loves those who are happy and carefree, without bitchiness, bitterness or regret. All of us need to work on reigniting our passion and desire as they are the burning fires that will change our make-up at a cellular level.

NinjaNewsflash

HARD TRAINING, EASY COMBAT
A healthy body begins with 'minding' your health. Training hard is important because it makes everything else in life more manageable. When you build up resilience through pushing the limits of your body, and experience pain and growth in the dojang or gym, then whatever combat you face in the outside world—stress, negativity, setbacks or disappointment—will be more easily defeated.

Tiff's Tip

Exercise and 'nude' foods are great medicine, cleansing the body and releasing feel-good endorphins.

Reconnect with energy

Weight is changeable. I think of excess weight as bad energy, which lurks in the heart and in the body. When emotional stress, negative influences and destructive people encroach on your life, the weight stacks on. But weight is fluid: it can go away, but also—all-too-often—come back. If you concentrate solely on the kilos, the fat will return. You need to focus your life around health, which means growing good energy in your relationships and in your home; using quality nutrition to cleanse the negative energy built up in your body; and exercising positive and self-nourishing thoughts to purge any detrimental energy in your mind.

If your goal is to lose weight, weigh yourself and write it down. You can't improve what you haven't measured. If your goal is to lower your cholesterol or blood pressure, have your cholesterol or blood pressure measured and write it down. You have to know where you are, as well as where you want to go, if you're going to get there. The first step is accepting the present truth.

Visualisation is a powerful tool: what you believe is what you will achieve. Picture yourself sitting at a table and only selecting foods that add health and vitality to your body. Visualise yourself participating in activities that enhance life and provide energy. Picture how free you will feel when eating pure, raw foods. Imagine life with real and lasting health. Take time each day to do this—do it at night after reading your warrior scrolls. It's a great and ancient mental and emotional exercise: I've found that once you believe something, with a real sense of certainty down deep in your core, it will almost always become true.

Work on your own warrior cry, which can be repeated to make you feel powerful and help you make stronger choices. Choose words that inspire you.

Just remember, there's no such thing as 'perfect'—perfection doesn't exist and if we set ourselves an unrealistic standard we'll feel we've failed and the negative cycle of self-loathing and weight gain will continue. We must accept ourselves, as we are, in any given moment. Through bad times and good times (a kilo of weight gain, a spate of pimples, a new relationship or burgeoning career), our self-love must be as unconditional and accepting, as free, fearless and limitless, as the love we are capable of giving others—without demands, comparisons or competition.

You are a gift to your body; you can make it stronger or weaker simply in the way you communicate with yourself. Your relationship with yourself is what shapes your future. Your identity is your destiny. How you see yourself is the person you will become. Toxic self-talk, like junk food, is a destructive habit. To change your circumstances you must first change your inner voice. Every second of every minute of every hour of every day, make sure you stand guard as a warrior at the gates to your mind.

NinjaNewsflash

RELAXATION IS RECOVERY

Weight loss happens when you are recovering. Those muscle fibres that were torn apart during exercise rebuild during recovery and the chemistry in your body rebalances so that you can burn fat more efficiently all day. Your body heals and changes during downtime, which is why it is so important to self-nurture and recover.

WARRIOR SCROLLS

Your mind contains a goal-seeking mechanism—once you have programmed a thought or desire into your subconscious it will work together with your conscious mind to steer you towards attaining it, whether positive or negative.

Until you put your goals in writing they exist only in the 'thinking' world, so put them in writing to make them exist in the 'doing' world as well. Post-its make the best warrior scrolls. I plaster power Post-its everywhere: my bedroom walls, bathroom mirror, fridge, car dashboard, TV. They remind me of what I want to achieve and who I already am—a warrior. Use these ninja mind tricks:

Detail your destiny

Be specific about what your life will be like once you've achieved your goal. Let your imagination explode. If your goal is eating 'naked' (see page 18), write in detail what your naked meals will look like and what you will be able to do with all the energy you will have. Then put this in an envelope to read when you need encouragement and motivation.

Brief your belief

Capture your goal in one sentence. For instance, you might write 'I choose only to eat nude foods (see page 18) in order to honour my body, to give vitality to my organs and cells and to increase my energy to play with my kids and, in the future, to play with my grandchildren'.

Write here and now

Remember to use 'I' next to each goal. Write in the present tense. Your subconscious mind responds only to commands that are personal, positive, active and immediate.

Journal your gratitude

Ask yourself, 'What have I made happen in my life that was once a dream?' What you believe, you will achieve. Fit people get fitter and rich people get richer because they focus on what they have, not what they're lacking. Your success in life will largely be determined by how clear you are about what it is you really, really want. Gratitude journaling is the best way to keep your focus positive and centred.

Revisit your habits

We are all creatures of habit—at work, at home, in relationships—and these habits dictate our thoughts and feelings. But sometimes our habits don't support our goals in life. The habit of complaining, of telling yourself you're not good enough, of eating when you're not hungry—these are all bad habits that have been conditioned over a long period of time and won't help you become a powerful weightloss warrior. Habits are a set of choices, the same ones made again and again until they become routine. Habits create outcomes: your body, your thoughts, your life are all the result of habits. They can build you the best or worst life, offer mediocrity or magnificence. You can blame habits, ignore habits, fight habits or, with focus and discipline, you can train habits to be on your side.

Create great habits and they will create a whole new you.

On your warrior journey to self-awareness it's important to become aware of your habits sooner rather than later. It is too late to re-evaluate your habit of smoking when you are diagnosed with lung cancer. You must stop the habits that hurt, keep the habits that support you in your journey, and start the habit that will help you grow.

The creation of a winning warrior habit requires two things: devotion and constant and never-ending improvement. Along the way you must celebrate mistakes—making mistakes is how we learn. Recognising them is how we know we're getting somewhere. Losing weight is all about making mistakes; after all, you're getting to know your body again (and again, as it changes shape and size), and the science of weight loss has a considerable margin for error. On our journey, don't burn your belt and give up just because you fall into temptation, make a mistake or bad decision. Ninjas are human too! When you are a healthy and fit black belt weightloss warrior there will be no mistake you can eat, no training you can miss, that would ruin your hard work. Listen to your body, learn from your mistakes, and navigate your way back to the warrior path.

We are what we repeatedly do: to create a habit you must embrace repetition. It is not only regime that changes lives but also routine. Repetition begins with a quality of focus. Weightloss warriors have a clear focus and know their desired outcome. They begin battle with an end in mind. What do you really desire? Clear goals deliver clearer outcomes. It makes it hard to hit your target if you're throwing ninja stars blindfolded.

You must also have passion. Emotionally engage with what you are focusing on to create a winning habit. Emotions drive commitment. The more powerful you feel about your goal, the harder it will be to stray from it. If you feel exercise is painful, too hard or embarrassing, then you'll never pursue it long-term because it's our natural instinct to avoid pain and pursue pleasure—which will then be staying at home and doing Couch Karate (TV on, TV off). But if you anchor—by remembering and emphasising—the feelings of pleasure, power, wellness and energy that exercise gives you, you'll become addicted to it because of the way it nourishes your human needs of self-love and connection, variety and growth.

Winning warrior habits are created out of repetition and devotion.

NinjaNewsflash
CREATE YOUR INNER DOJANG

Self-control is hard. One of the few things we can control in life is how well we treat ourselves through healthy choices and empowering actions. Once you gain control of how you feel, how you eat, how you think, how you move, then you will feel more in control when it comes to the outside world.

Tiff's Tip

Own it, don't clone it.
Stop comparing yourself to
other people—everyone has
something that someone else
wants whether it's fuller
breasts, clearer skin or
more or less hair!

Review your support

No one ever said you have to set—and stick to—goals on your own. Who can help you? Surround yourself with a ninja army of activists and enthusiasts and you will become accountable by being accountable to others. Measure your goals with a partner, a coach, a friend or colleague. Team up with people who are striving for the same goal: if you are trying to quit smoking, surround yourself with non-smokers, if you are trying to get fit, surround yourself with energetic people, if you are trying to break into a particular industry, surround yourself with people who are passionate about that industry too. Make new friends and networks of friends who will help you get to where you want to be. Everyone needs a tribe, and the right friends could make all the difference when it comes to losing those kilos.

Camaraderie can help create a sense of urgency. You are committed. Now is the time for action. Do something that will move you closer to your target: it could be a tiny step, like going for a walk, or a giant leap, such as going to the kitchen and throwing away all your packaged, processed, lifeless so-called food.

Weightloss warriors must create urgency, immerse themselves in their new habits and take action!

NinjaNewsflash

TAKE TIME TO TURN OFF
Advanced technology means we're always connected, always bombarded. We can work anywhere, anytime, with screens that fit in our pockets, but working more than 40 hours a week doubles women's risk of depression and increases men's risk by 33 per cent. Don't make yourself a walking heart attack. Switch off your iPhone and sit with yourself for a while. Relax and reboot. Like all the appliances we lug around, our batteries need recharging too.

MAKE OVER YOUR MIND

Trade 'hiding' for 'seeking': find out why you're overweight. Ask the hard questions, and then do the hard yards to change your habits. Weight isn't just physical, it's emotional.

Trade an 'I can't have this' mindset for a 'Look what I can still have' one. Make a list of everything you *can* eat so you don't feel deprived.

Give up thinking weight loss is magical. Say: 'Losing weight starts with me!'

Apply the same determination to weight loss that you would to anything else: there are setbacks in careers and relationships but we don't give up on them. Why give up on health and happiness so easily?

Trade emotional eating for soul searching—journaling is the best way to let out your emotions.

Swap sabotage for support.

Stop asking 'Am I skinny enough?' and instead say 'How's my health?' Weightloss warriors focus on nurturing the mind, body and spirit.

Biggest Loser contestants have to be honest with their starting weight, weighing-in and confronting their fears in front of everybody they know. Publicly announcing your weight and pledging never to return to it can be a powerful act of confession and commitment.

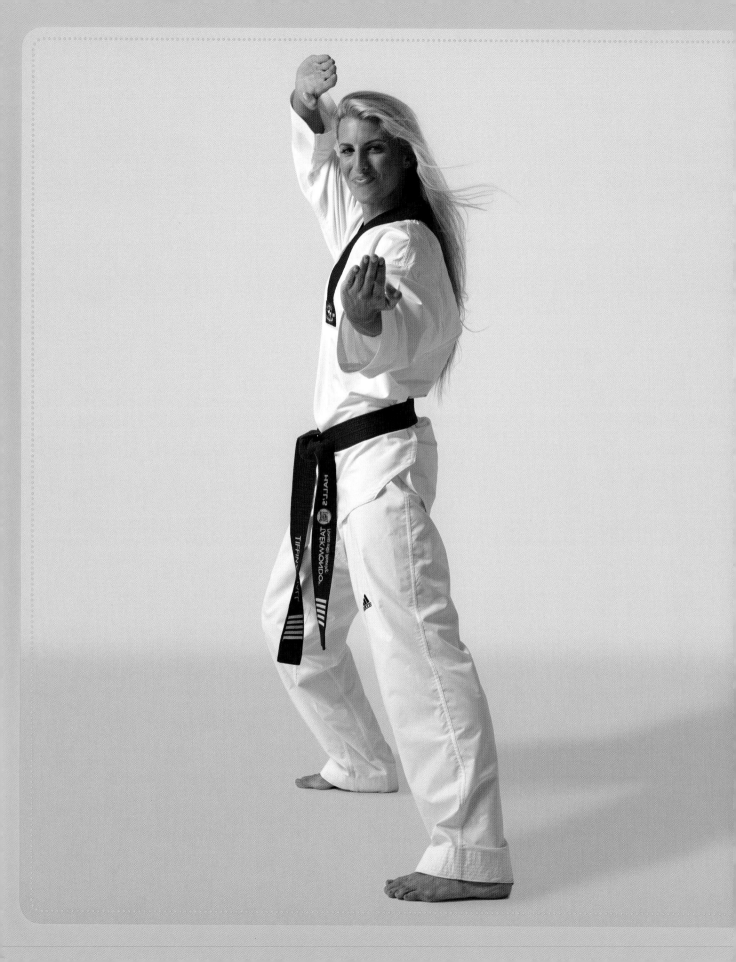

Yellow belt: Warrior energy

'DIET IS A FOUR-LETTER WORD WHEN IT COMES TO RETRAINING YOUR MIND, REBALANCING YOUR BODY AND RESTORING YOUR HORMONES'

Eat naked

The first thing a warrior must learn is how the world works. In our case, as weightloss warriors, this means understanding how *you* work (starting with your mind) and then, most importantly, moving on to how food works in your body. Oh, yeah, and how and why the diet and food-manufacturing industries do what they do.

Don't be bewildered by any of the information here, don't get confused by the lists of ingredients on packaging or the science of metabolism. If you need it short and sweet, just remember to eat 'close to the source'. Is this food pretty much how it appears in nature? ('No' to Tim Tams, soft drink, pizza and white bread; 'Yes' to brown rice, vegies and meat.)

Don't eat ingredients you don't have in the pantry: cellulose? xanthan? ethoxylated glycerides? If you don't cook with these ingredients, why let others cook with them for you? We haven't been ingesting them long enough to know what side effects they could have.

The answer is simple: eat naked. I do. I LOVE IT: nude food rules!

Nude foods will harmonise your hormones, speed up your metabolism, cleanse and alkalise your body. (Alkaline tissue holds twenty times more oxygen than acidic tissue.) It's difficult to get sick when you're eating naked foods that make your body alkaline: germs, bacteria, viruses, fungi and diseases need acid to thrive. Acids are formed through stress, negative emotions and eating fake food that's processed and package with not enough vitamins and minerals.

NinjaMove

DON'T *BUY* JUNK FOOD
Manufacturers are making formerly expensive and hard-to-make treats so cheap and easy we're eating them every day. If you only eat fries, rocky road, burgers and ice-cream you make yourself, you'll eat them less often. And burn calories cooking! Bake a cake—enjoy it: if you know what's in the stuff you cook, you'll know what stuff is going into your body. In fact, it won't really be 'junk' food!

WARRIOR CHEMISTRY

Fad diets not only change the way your body burns fat, they also change your chemistry so your body produces more fat-storing enzymes to save up fat for the next time you diet. Even worse, fad diets increase your appetite! In starvation mode your body tries to trick you into eating by intensifying your cravings. Every time you reduce your food intake, your brain immediately switches on hormones that make you want to eat more while those that normally make you feel full drop off. No matter how disciplined you are, you won't be able to fight hormonal hunger—which is why when you go off a fad diet you fly off it with a vengeance.

Tiff's Tip

When choosing food ask yourself: 'Would my great-granny recognise it?' If she wouldn't, neither will your body.

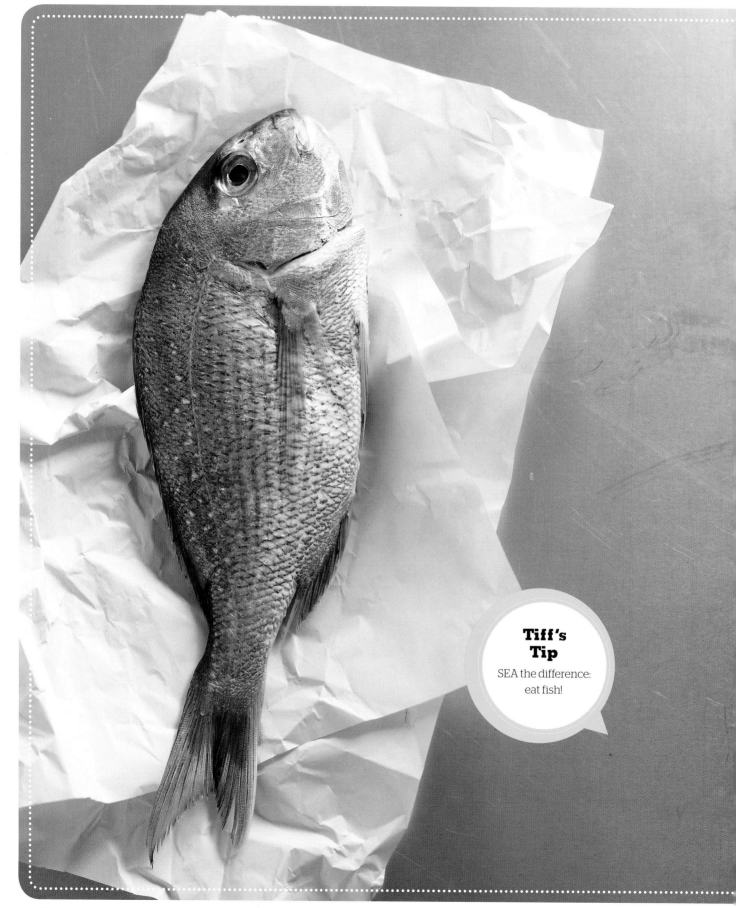

Tiff's Tip

SEA the difference:
eat fish!

PROTEIN POINTERS

Choose a variety of proteins each day. Try yoghurt for breakfast; beans for lunch; cottage cheese as a snack; grilled salmon for dinner.

As you age and muscle is depleted women need more calcium. Choose two servings of calcium-rich protein from low-sugar dairy proteins every day.

Fish is low-calorie, high-protein and heart-healthy, as well as rich in omega-3 fatty acid, vitamin E and selenium.

Free-range meats and eggs are best—free of antibiotics and growth hormones with less saturated fat.

Avoid processed meats. Not only are they high in fat, they contain sodium nitrites, which react with foods in your stomach to form potentially cancer-causing chemicals. Very acidic too!

Food fashion

Like most chicks I'm a sucker for fashion. I'm never far away from those glossy magazines showcasing the latest trends. But some trends hurt and I'm not talking about blisters from Jimmy Choo shoes; I'm talking about food fashion. There's no point adopting food habits that are in vogue simply because someone you don't know tried them once. One size fits all may work for some dresses but when it comes to health, one-off fad diets won't fit you and your body type. Every metabolism is hormonally unique: you can't eat the same stuff as everyone else because it won't balance out *your* chemistry. The fact is one-fad-fits-all will make you unfit in terms of health, hormones, self-esteem and relationships—especially your relationship with food.
Don't get angry with carbs; don't kick fat out the house; don't break up with your favourite desserts and swear you'll never see them again.

Don't even try on the latest diet: be fashion forward and opt for healthy long-term warrior habits instead. Fad diets are out of fashion—but unlike a fashion faux pas they're a trend that can do significant long-term damage. Losing weight by starving your body results in hormonal damage. Starvation diets are catabolic, which means they encourage your body to eat itself, to break down your muscles for fuel. That's because muscles take more calories to run, so your body will ditch them knowing it will then need fewer calories to function. Clever, huh?

Without muscle your metabolism is slower so when you do start eating normally again your hormones will have changed to store fat at super-fast speed. When you cut your food intake your body sets off an alarm called the 'starvation response'; this tells your body to hold onto fat stores and conserve energy by slowing down your metabolism. Back in the caveman days, when we didn't know where our next meal was coming from, storing energy kept us alive and allowed the human species to survive.

NinjaNewsflash
IT'S NOT (ONLY) YOUR FAULT
Between 1977 and 1996 the average cheeseburger grew in size by 25 per cent. In that same time the average bag of pretzels grew by 93 calories (389 kJ).

Let's not sugar-coat the truth; the success of the sixty-billion-dollar diet industry thrives on the inevitable failure of the Diet Devotee. The diet industry understands the starvation response all too well, knowing you may lose weight initially, but when you 'break' (which you will) you'll regain the weight you lost plus more. The next time you go on a fad diet your body will be armed with an extra 5 kilos! One sure way to keep a Dedicated Dietess devoted is to make her fatter. Ninety-nine per cent of all fad diets fail, yet the diet industry has never been in such great shape—unlike us!

It doesn't matter who you are or what you do, you will never outsmart your body. Most women, right now, are on a diet that is making them fat. Australians spend more than a million dollars a day on weight-loss products, investing money, health and energy in the latest pill, package or promise that's being pushed by big, slick marketing campaigns. Aren't you sick of it? Sick of not fitting into those jeans; sick of feeling self-conscious on the beach; sick of battling your yoyoing weight? Diets have failed me and they're failing you. The dieting industry has failed us, so let's get our ninja on and take back control like the warriors we are!

NinjaNewsflash
ASSASSINS ON YOUR SIDE
Vegies are like little assassins in the body, eliminating carcinogens before they cause genetic damage and helping to restore balance to your hormones. Their fibre fills you up and can increase fat burn by 30 per cent.

Food friends and foes

To make food work for you, you have to be able to distinguish your enemies from your allies—the same as any warrior would, going into battle.

Protein packs a punch

Protein provides the building blocks for the body to construct and repair tissue such as muscle, hair, nails and skin. Protein is the raw construction material for your body's cells; next to water it is the most abundant substance in your body. Protein breaks down into amino acids and also makes enzymes, antibodies and hormones. Protein helps you feel fuller for longer, keeps your insulin levels stable, works as a natural diuretic, and burns off a lot of itself during the process of digestion.

Some protein-rich foods are dairy; beans and lentils; quinoa; tempeh; fish, and—yup, you guessed it!—meat (though always remove the skin from chicken to reduce the fat, and it's best to only eat red meat twice a week as it's high in saturated fats).

Chew these carb corrections

Carbohydrates are quick energy for the body, which breaks them down into glucose and stores it as glycogen or, if not used, as fat. The muscles hold 80 per cent of the body's glycogen stores while the remaining 20 per cent are stored in the liver. The body stores, on average, 2000 calories (8,372 kJ) in its muscles as 500 grams of glycogen for energy production, whereas even a lean person will have 100,000-plus calories (418,600 kJ) in the form of stored fat. So glycogen is a limited fuel source whereas fat is not. The body can't afford to run out of glycogen so when exercise extends it begins to burn fat. You'll get the best burn after 20 minutes of exercise, once glycogen stores are depleted. When your body is low on glycogen it has no choice but to burn fat. That's why some people prefer to exercise before breakfast as the body's glycogen stores are at their lowest. The body generally has enough glycogen to last for two hours of physical activity.

Avoid the SHAMwich!

Eating white bread is like chewing cardboard coated in sugar or eating papier-mâché. White bread is my pet hate! It's bleached with chemicals such as oxide of nitrogen, chlorine, chloride, nitrosyl and benzoyl peroxide mixed with various other chemicals to make it white. When the flour is bleached in the factory, all the good nutrients such as unsaturated fatty acids, vitamin E, calcium, iron, magnesium and other nutrients are also stripped out. Essentially, when white bread is made, the good bits like dietary fibre are removed and bad bits are added—such as sugars and salt. Eating white bread can cause a rise in blood sugar levels due to its high-GI carbohydrates, raise the levels of bad cholesterol in your bloodstream, and can cause your metabolism to slow down due to its lack of dietary fibre. Conclusion: white is not alright!

Make sure the first ingredient listed on any carbohydrate label is 'whole wheat', 'wholemeal', or 'wholegrain'. 'Wheat flour' means enriched flour with some whole wheat added. Never trust the word 'enriched' on a label when buying pasta or bread. Foods made with processed white flour are low in fibre: meaning nutrients have been stripped and replaced synthetically. A good rule of thumb when selecting bread is to look for 100 per cent wholemeal or wholegrain flour or stone-ground flour. (Stone-ground flour means the whole grain is crushed between moving stones, so you're still getting the nutritional value of the whole grain.)

Choose breads with 2 or more grams of fibre per serving. Choose high-fibre, which has around 45 (188 kJ) calories per slice of bread. Flaxseeds (also called linseeds) and pumpkin seeds all offer great nutritional benefits and always check the sodium content and if sugars have been added to the bread.

NinjaNewsflash

WHOLEGRAINS ARE BEST
Brown rice is higher in vitamins and fibre than white rice, which has been stripped of its husk, germ and bran layers during processing. Rolled oats are more nutritious than instant oats. When grains are put through the process of refinement, the important nutrients are taken out and all that remains is the starchy interior loaded with carbohydrates and not much else.

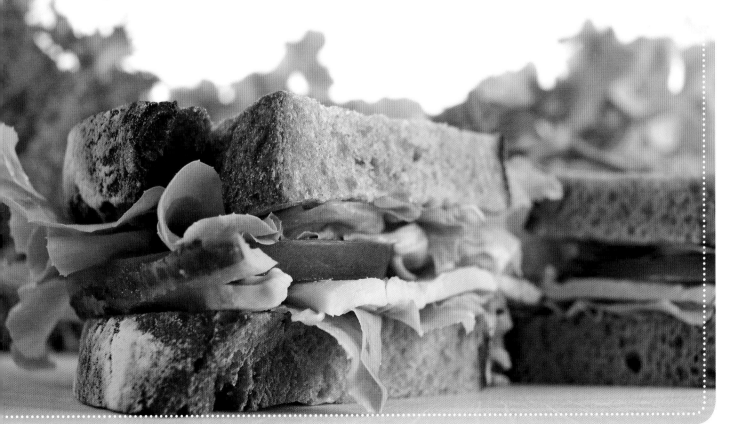

CONTROL YOUR CRAVINGS

Stomp out overeating by eating every 4 hours, adhering to my 3, 2, 1 rule. That is, eat three well-portioned healthy home-cooked meals a day, two healthy snacks and at least a litre of water to fire up your metabolism.

Crunch cravings by eating the right food combinations. Focus on palm-sized portions of protein (fish, chicken, turkey, lean meats, eggs), at least 20 per cent good fats (avocados, raw nuts, flaxseed oils) and fill up on salads and vegies.

Exercise mind control and really identify the difference between hunger and hurt. Take a deep breath and ask yourself if you are hungry or just upset? If you're upset, address those feelings—don't eat your emotions.

Train your sweet tooth with exercise: suppressing appetite is one of the many benefits of physical exercise. If you're lusting for sweets, a 20–30 minute brisk walk will hunger-proof you against their delicious demands.

Resist the hunger ambush by making sure you're not thirsty. Often when we feel voraciously hungry we're actually thirsty. When your body is dehydrated hormones trigger hunger sensations to get you to eat so you can absorb water from the food. How smart is that! If you've been binging, food increases the thickness of your blood and your body senses the need to dilute it. The worst thing you can do for hunger-thirst is drink soft drinks or alcohol. So if you're more hungry than usual, increase your fluids, take twenty sips of water and if it's hunger-thirst that will work as an appetite suppressant.

Take time out from binging when you're eating everything and anything because your hunger hormones and cravings have kicked in. Break for 20 minutes. It takes 20 minutes for your brain to receive the 'I'm full' signal from your stomach. If after 20 minutes you're still hungry, go for a 5 minute walk!

A good night's sleep is integral to appetite control. Sleep deprivation disrupts the boss appetite hormones. In order to restore its chemical balance your body will crave sugary foods to give you an instant hit of serotonin, which you deprived yourself of through lack of sleep. If you have trouble sleeping exercise is the best way to regulate your body clock. Activity increases oxygen in the blood and circulation to wake you up fresh so that by bedtime you will sleep soundly.

GO NUTS!

Add nuts to muesli, salads, pasta, homemade breads, stir-fries and savoury muffins to suppress appetite. Use nut spreads on rice cakes, wholegrain breads and celery sticks. Sprinkle chopped nuts in oats, on natural yoghurt or cottage cheese. Add ground-nut mixes such as LSA to smoothies. Cashews go great guns in casseroles. Walnuts and pecans peak in baked goods. I always have bags of almonds, pumpkin seeds, pine nuts, brazil nuts in my bag as emergency snacks.

Almonds are high in protein, calcium and magnesium and lower cholesterol.

Brazil nuts have the highest selenium content of all nuts. Selenium is a powerful antioxidant that is thought to prevent cancer.

Cashews are great for glowing eyes—rich in minerals and mono-unsaturated fats, good fats that make you thin.

Macadamias are another cholesterol buster.

Pecans are packed with power: over nineteen vitamins and minerals.

Walnuts are the greatest source of omega-3 fats, which are awesome for your heart.

Tiff's Tip

Eat the low-calorie
proportion of your meal first—
salad, vegies and soup. Eat slowly.
Eat the meats and starches last.
By the time you get to them
you should be full enough
to eat smaller portions.

For the carb-anxious out there, relax. Carbohydrates don't make you fat—*processed* carbohydrates make you fat. Eating wholegrain carbs like rolled oats, wholegrain bread and wholegrain pastas will aid you in losing weight by helping absorb protein into your system and fuelling your body for exercise. Your body can only store 1200 calories (5,023 kJ) of carbohydrates (as glycogen) at a time, the rest gets stored as fat. But 1200 calories (5,023kJ) of carbs will start burning in the first 90 seconds of exercise.

The lie of low-GI

Glycaemic index is a measure of the degree to which any given food spikes blood sugar, similar to how different woods might burn on a fire. Some foods (high-GI) burn very quickly, like paper, other foods (low–GI) burn slowly for hours, like hardwood sleepers. But 'low-GI' can be another misleading label: low-GI foods may release energy more slowly, so you don't peak and crash as you do with foods high in glucose, but this index was designed to help people manage type 2 diabetes, not help us lose weight. Food that has a large percentage of fat usually has a lower GI rating. So does fructose, since it's invisible to our pancreas.

Some low-GI foods are good for you—I certainly recommend switching to multigrain bread when you discover your cereal is over one-quarter sugar! But many manufacturers are using the 'invisible fat' loophole to gain marketing advantage. Almost any chocolate-based product will be low-GI because of its high-fat and low-fructose content (not to mention a Pizza Hut Stuffed Crust BBQ Meatlovers)—even if marketers aren't courageous enough to label chocolate bars low-GI yet. If you're not diabetic, use your tongue. Sweet foods, even if low-GI, shouldn't be eaten often.

Why we need good fats

If you want to get rid of the fat on your body, put some more in your mouth. It's true: good fats help you lose weight. We need that fat to think, grow and absorb essential vitamins and antioxidants. Fat makes foods taste wonderful and helps us feel satisfied. Healthy fats help our hearts and feed our brains.

NinjaNewsflash

JUST SAY 'NO'!

If you think a sneaky biscuit here and there won't hurt, remind yourself that two cream biscuits at a morning tea and two in an office meeting can deliver up to 420 calories (1,758 kJ), 28 grams of fructose and 12.5 grams of fat. This means that besides dumping 12.5 grams of fat into my arteries, those little snacks deliver 112 invisible calories (469 kJ) in JUST ONE DAY! A kilo of body fat is 7000 calories (29,302 kJ), so if I snacked this way for 2 months I'd gain a kilo alone without my body ever having noticed me eating anything at all.

HOW GOOD FATS WILL GET YOU THIN

No-fat or low-fat diets trigger the starvation response.

No fat causes fluctuations in blood sugar. Fat slows the release of carbohydrates into the bloodstream, so when large amounts of simple and refined carbohydrates are eaten alone they rapidly shoot into the bloodstream, creating a large spike in blood sugar.

No fat causes greater insulin release. When your blood sugar spikes, your pancreas releases a lot of insulin to bring your blood sugar back to normal levels. Moderate amounts of insulin are necessary to make muscles grow, but large amounts of insulin cause fat storage and prevent fat burning.

No fat causes hormone-related hunger and cravings. You can't fight hormonal hunger; it will always drive you to the fridge.

Eating good fats, such as polyunsaturated and mono-unsaturated fats, increases your metabolic rate and helps to burn body fat faster.

'The health ninja one-second, foolproof, long-lasting weight-loss diet: decide now—before you turn the page—to go off all fad diets forever!'

Tiff's Tip

Weightloss warriors, if you
want to be super hardcore, toss
out the bread slices and wrap your
burger or sandwich fillings in a
leaf or two of cos lettuce.
Or eat it with a fork!

Fat is one of the three classes of nutrients (along with proteins and carbohydrates) that we can't live without. There are three types of fat: triglycerides, cholesterol and phospholipids. The reason we have fat is to provide the body with energy—many people are surprised to find out that fat actually contains more energy (calories) than protein and carbohydrates. Fat also serves other important purposes—it helps our bodies absorb vitamins A, D, E and K.

Fat is sustained energy, providing cushioning and insulation for the body, as well as being involved in brain function, nerve transmission and hormone production. It's eventually broken down into free fatty acids through the process of digestion. Once fat is digested it's transported to the cells for conversion or is stored in the fat cells. The average 70 kg body carries 90,000 (376,740 kJ) to 135,000 calories (565,110 kJ) of fat: that's 10–15 kilos. (The fat that's most dangerous is that stored around your stomach: visceral fat.) The average person has fifty billion fat cells. Fat cells are like storage tanks of energy for later use and look like water balloons. These balloons can be flat or full. Fat cells can multiply. And binge eating stimulates baby fat cells to sprout.

Fit people are better fat-burning machines. It would be fantastic if we could use 100 per cent fat as energy but intensity and duration affects the fuels we use. To burn fat, forget slow, moderate exercise and hit the intensity!

And keep putting that good fat into your body—on a fat-loss diet 10 per cent of your calories should be good fats. Today, fat is no longer seen as the enemy when it comes to healthy weight loss. So make sure you know your fat friends—those that increase your metabolic rate and help you burn stored fat faster—from your fat foes!

FORGET FAD DIETS FOREVER

Fad dieting is the greatest risk factor in developing an eating disorder. Sixty-eight per cent of 15-year-old girls in Australia are on a fad diet right now. Eight per cent of these girls are dieting severely. Adolescent girls who diet moderately are five times more likely to develop an eating disorder than those who don't diet, and those who diet severely are eighteen times more likely.

Dieting is disordered eating and disordered eating is the first clinical sign of an eating disorder. Girls are dieting at younger and younger ages. The Eating Disorders Foundation of Victoria reported a 200 per cent increase in eating disorders in children aged 7 to 10 years old in 2010.

We're caught in a vicious cycle: the fatter we get from fad dieting, the more obsessed we become with being thin, and the younger we all start dieting. Australian women who start dieting before the age of fifteen are more likely to experience depression, binge eating, purging, low iron levels and menstrual irregularities. Women who diet frequently (that is, have been on a diet more than five times) are 75 per cent more likely to experience depression.

If you're mindlessly following someone else's diet you've seen in a magazine or on TV then stop. You don't want to lose 5 kilos five times over; you want to lose 5 kilos forever. One of the hardest battles a weightloss warrior must fight is killing the diet mentality and replacing it with a black belt mindset. You will only win the battle within when you understand that starvation does not equal fat loss.

NinjaMove

LOAD UP TO TRIM DOWN!
Eat more mono-unsaturated fats like extra virgin olive oil, almonds, avocados, canola oil, cashews, macadamia nuts, peanuts, pistachios and polyunsaturated fats such as flaxseeds and pumpkin seeds, as well as salmon, cabbage, cauliflower, mackerel, soybean oil, steamed broccoli, tofu and walnuts. Pop a cap of good fats with fish oils—up to 1000 milligrams a day.

Fat friends

Mono-unsaturated fats reduce blood pressure, help brain function and improve arterial function. Thirty per cent of your fat intake should be mono-unsaturated. Mono-unsaturated fats are found in olive and canola oils, flaxseeds, avocados and raw nuts such as pistachios, walnuts, cashews and almonds.

One tablespoon of flaxseed oil or Udo's Choice Oil Blend can fix you up with essential fatty acids for the day.

Polyunsaturated fats are also really good for you and come in two forms—omega-3 and omega-6. Polyunsaturated fats can help lower cholesterol and reduce the risk of heart disease. Omega-3 fats are found in fish and omega-6 fats in oils such as safflower, sesame and soybean oils, as well as some nuts such as brazil nuts.

Foods such as salmon, trout and sardines are a fabulous source of fatty acids.

NinjaNewsflash

WHERE SUGAR HIDES

Like the devil, sugar answers to many names: brown rice syrup, cane juice, caramel, carob syrup, chocolate syrup, cinnamon sugar, coarse sugar, coconut sugar, corn syrup, corn syrup solids, date syrup, demerara, dextran, dextrose, diatase, disaccharide, erythritol, ethyl maltol, fructose, fruit juice concentrate, fruit syrup, galacatose, glucose, glucose solids, glycerol, golden brown sugar, golden caster sugar, golden icing sugar, golden sugar, golden syrup, granulated sugar, grape sugar, grape sweetener, high-fructose corn syrup, high-maltose corn syrup, honey, invert sugar, lactose, levulose, malt, malt extract, maltose, mannitol, molasses, monosaccharide, refiner's syrup, rice extract, sorbitol, sucrose.

Fat foes

These fats have the lowest thermic effect of all nutrients, increasing their health risks. This means it takes less heat to digest fat than it does carbohydrates or protein. It only takes 3 per cent of the calories in fat to digest and utilise it, whereas it takes nearly 30 per cent of the calories in protein foods to burn them off and absorb them.

Trans fats (also called 'trans fatty acids') are by far the worst of the fats—they're pure evil! Trans fats cause bloating, clogging and turn your body into a fat-storing machine. Although trans fats can be found in small amounts in natural foods, such as beef, lamb and dairy, usually these ones are unsaturated fats that have been processed in order to act like saturated fats. This process is called hydrogenation. Partial hydrogenation is an industrial process that makes healthy oil into unhealthy oil in order to make oil more solid, provide longer shelf-life in baked products, give longer fry-life for cooking oils, and a certain texture in your mouth. Trans fats can increase your body's 'bad' cholesterol and decrease its 'good' cholesterol levels. It also amplifies the risk of heart attacks and heart disease.

Foods high in trans fats include deep-fried fast foods, heavily manufactured baked and pastry goods and shortening—all of which are on the naughty ninja list!

Saturated fats are fats that are solid at room temperature, such as those found in animal products (meats and dairy) or some plant sources (coconut milk and palm oil). Consumption of saturated fat should be kept low, especially for adults, as it's linked to an increased risk of heart disease and unhealthy cholesterol levels.

Foods such as butter, cream and cheese contain high levels of saturated fats, as do heavily manufactured and pre-packaged foods such as pastries, cakes and biscuits. Fatty cuts of meat, chicken with the skin left on, and processed meats such as salami are also high in bad fats.

The real enemy: Phantom fat

Fat makes you fat, right? Fat-free foods are healthy, right? WRONG!

When we eat fat, or protein, our upper intestine releases a hormone called cholecystokinin (CCK). CCK tells our brain to suppress hunger and make us feel full. CCK is our internal calorie counter. So if CCK is monitoring our fat intake and telling our brain we're full, why are we still fat? Because something is slipping past the keeper. Something we can eat in unlimited quantities, that never makes us feel full. Not protein. Not complex carbohydrate. Not fat. SUGAR!

(Remember 'fat-free' usually means 'sugar-loaded'.)

Carbohydrates such as grains, breads and pasta are almost entirely glucose, but sugar is only half glucose. The other half is fructose. Eating fructose is like eating invisible fat because it slips past your body's defences: your gut will process as much fructose as you put in your mouth, there's no limit. Fructose bypasses our appetite-control systems and jumps a critical step in our metabolism that would ordinarily stop our arteries filling up with circulating fat. Eating fat still puts fat in our arteries, but we have a built-in control to stop us eating too much fat. There's no such thing for fructose.

It's the sweet stuff that causes weight gain. Eating sugar pumps up your appetite and is addictive. Sugar hits up the same neurotransmitters that activate the brain's pleasure state as addictive drugs such as including morphine and heroin. Without it you'd have withdrawals: depression, anxiety, lethargy, mood change. Make no mistake, sugar is a drug. Addictiveness is exacerbated when sugar is absorbed on an empty stomach, so rethink the sweet coffee instead of breakfast next time.

Tiff's Tip

Fat comes in the form of friends and foes—heroes that make you healthy and villains that make you fat—but there's no such thing as good sugar.

HIGH-FRUCTOSE FOODS (PER 100 GRAMS)

Honey—40.1 grams	Sweet pickles—9 grams
Sultanas—30 grams	Grapes—8 grams
Figs—29.6 grams	Pineapple—7.2 grams
Dates—19.5 grams	Tomato sauce—9 grams
Prune puree—13.8 grams	Regular coke—6.1 grams
Dried peaches—13.5 grams	Caffeine-free coke—6.1 grams
Apples—6 grams	Reduced-fat French dressing—12 grams
Pears—6.2 grams	Apple juice—5.6 grams
Tomato paste—6 grams	Dried apricots—12.5 grams

Marketers think they can fool you with the line 'contains only natural sugar', but the product in question may have been sweetened with honey. Yes, honey is better for you than cane sugar but it still contains 40 per cent fructose (compared to the 50 per cent in sugar). It's hardly gonna help you unleash your inner warrior! 'Natural sugar' is code for 'contains high levels of fructose'. Fruit juices are all natural sugars; cereals packed with sultanas and raisins are full of 'natural sugar' so they don't need added sugar.

'Fat-free' plays the same trick, directly translating to 'high fructose'. Low-fat means sugar packed, salt stuffed or artificially sweetened. Food industry honchos know that if they go on long enough about bad fats, you won't notice the even more evil sugar. Next time you're at the supermarket compare the sugar content of a low-fat food item with its full-fat equivalent. I guarantee it will contain more sugar. It's a LOL moment when I see marshmallows or licorice advertised as 99 per cent fat free—they're 100 per cent sugar. Chocolate is one-third fat and actually better for you.

The worst sugar: Fructose

Eating large amounts of sugar increases the hormone cortisol, which is produced in the adrenal gland and is the stress hormone. Sugar temporarily increases blood pressure (for extra thinking) and blood sugar (for extra energy) and suppresses the body's immune system. This sugar high SHUTS DOWN fat burn.

We have an appetite control centre in our brain called the hypothalamus, which reacts to four major appetite hormones. Three of them (insulin, leptin and CCK) tell us when we've had enough to eat. Every morsel of food stimulates the release of one or more of the 'I'm stuffed!' hormones once we've had enough. But fructose is invisible to these hormones. Humans are the only mammal that gets obese and it's not because of fat, it's because we wipe ourselves out with sugar. Lions don't trim the fat off their prey; they eat the fat until they feel full and stop.

Fructose skips the fat-creation control mechanism in the liver that signals that you've had enough fat and protein. It is converted straight to fatty acids and then body fat without passing through any of the appetite-control centres (insulin or CCK). You burn 23 calories (96 kJ) to convert 100 calories (418 kJ) of protein or glucose into body fat. It only takes 2.5 (10 kJ) calories to convert 100 calories (418 kJ) of fatty acids into body fat. Guess what, even our fat cells are lazy! They'd rather store circulating fatty acids as fat than go to the trouble of converting glucose to body fat using insulin. Too much hard yakka! We can eat as much fructose as we fancy and never feel full—in fact, we'll feel hungrier.

Glucose is the form of energy you were designed to run on. Every cell in your body, every bacterium, every living thing on the earth uses glucose for energy. If you received your fructose only from vegetables and fruits (where it originates), as your great grandparents did, you'd consume about 15 grams per day, a far cry from the 73 grams the typical adolescent absorbs from sweetened drinks alone. In vegetables and fruits, sugar is mixed in with fibre, vitamins, minerals, enzymes, and beneficial phytonutrients, all of which moderate any negative metabolic effects.

NinjaNewsflash

THE *FAT* BOTTOM LINE

Fructose leads to increased belly fat, insulin resistance and metabolic syndrome. Weightloss warriors know that even the humble apple has the same amount of fructose as 2 teaspoons of sugar. Limiting sugar is the best way to regulate your metabolism since fructose subverts our appetite control and creates fat instantly!

There are two reasons fructose is the weightloss warrior's enemy. First, where glucose suppresses the hunger hormone ghrelin and stimulates leptin (which suppresses appetite), fructose has no effect on ghrelin and interferes with your brain's communication with leptin, resulting in overeating. Second, after eating fructose, 100 per cent of the metabolic weight rests on your liver, whereas with glucose your liver has to break down only 20 per cent. Every cell in your body, including your brain, utilises glucose so most of it is burned up immediately after you consume it. Fructose is turned into free fatty acids and triglycerides, which get stored as fat. Not only that but the fatty acids created during fructose metabolism accumulate as fat droplets in your liver and skeletal muscle tissues, causing insulin resistance and non-alcoholic fatty liver disease (NAFLD). Insulin resistance progresses to metabolic syndrome and type 2 diabetes.

Eat 120 calories (502 kJ) of glucose, and less than 1 calorie (4 kJ) is stored as fat; eat 120 calories (502 kJ) of fructose and 40 calories (167 kJ) are stored as fat. Consuming fructose is essentially consuming fat! The metabolism of fructose by your liver creates a long list of waste products and toxins, including a large amount of uric acid, which drives up blood pressure and causes gout. So if anyone tries to tell you 'sugar is sugar', not fat, they're obviously on some kind of high.

A tale of two sugars

When you think of sugar you probably picture the white stuff you stir into your coffee. Actually this is just one form of sugar, called sucrose, that's extracted from sugar cane. Technically sugar is a carbohydrate that occurs naturally in every fruit and vegetable. It's the major product of photosynthesis, the process by which plants transform the sun's energy into food.

You can think of sugars in two groups, those that occur naturally (such as fructose in fruit and lactose in milk and dairy products—but be aware that fructose can also be used as an added sugar: in some novelty beverages such as Bubble Tea; some energy bars; and some 'natural' packaged foods such as health-food store biscuits). Then there are added sugars, like those used in baking or coffee. Added sugar can take many different forms, from raw, brown, cane through to sucrose, glucose, fructose, malt, maltose, corn syrup, lactose, sorbitol, mannitol, honey, molasses, evaporated cane juice and barley malt extract.

Added sugars shouldn't make up more than 10 per cent of your total energy intake for the day, and many dietitians will recommend less than this. In a 2000 calorie-a-day (8,372 kJ) diet, 10 per cent is equal to about 50 grams, or 10 teaspoons of sugar. Unfortunately most Australians consume 30–40 teaspoons or more of refined sugar per day—far more than is healthy. Most of this comes from food products to which sugar has been added, such as soft drinks, confectionary and baked goods. A can of soft drink alone can contain up to 10 teaspoons of added sugar!

NinjaMove

WEANING OFF SUGAR

Eat breakfast: when you eat breakfast you prevent the drop in blood sugar that makes you crave sweet things later. Better still, opt for a fatty brekkie—a 'good fat' breakfast that is: avocado and tomato on rye toast with cinnamon, or eggs, or cottage cheese with shavings of nuts. Those will make you feel full all day, or at least until lunchtime!

Tiff's Tip

When it comes to sugar, cut out the sneaky stuff—the fat-free, sugar-loaded snacks—and replace them with 'naked' alternatives like carrots or red capsicums.

Get yourself to sugar rehab

It's a killer that there's no diet equivalent to wean us off biscuits—they're all low-fat and pure evil. (Remember, low-fat biscuits have even more sugar than regular bickies—being low-fat they must be stuffed full of even more sugar to get some taste into them). Whatever your weakness, when it comes to sugary snacks a weightloss warrior has to exercise self-control and simply go cold turkey. Whenever you see a sugary snack just say to yourself, 'I don't eat that'. Be positive. Personal. Use the present tense.

Remove the jar of biscuits and replace it with nuts; nuts will fill you up. They still contain a lot of calories but the difference is they're all being counted and you will soon feel full. The famous nut bloat will let you know!

In a nutshell, almonds are the best-absorbed source of vitamin E. Muscles crave vitamin E because the potent antioxidants help prevent free radical damage after exercise. When you first enter sweet rehab, your body will crave sugar. You'll be irritable, lethargic and headachy—you'll be like any other addict coming off drugs. But soon your body will crave sugar less as it regains its insulin sensitivity.

NinjaNewsflash

NO SAFE SUGAR SUBSTITUTES?
Scientists continue to search for the perfect sugar substitute but recent media coverage questions whether these chemical concoctions can really be healthy: aspartame can trigger head pain (experts believe the phenylalanine in aspartame has a negative impact on neurotransmitters) and HFCS has been found to increase the risk of metabolic syndrome. Many nutritionists agree you'll be healthier and more satisfied eating a bit of post-lunch chockie than feasting on artificially sweetened foods all day.

WHEN SUGARS AIN'T SUGARS

Sugarine is saccharin, your granny's sugar substitute, which was discovered in 1879 and is the result of a chemical reaction that produces methyl anthranilate (yum!). It contains just .01 calories (.04 kJ) per teaspoon versus sugar's 15 calories (62 kJ), yet is 300 times sweeter than the natural stuff. The downside of saccharin, used in products like Diet Pepsi and even some toothpastes, is obvious from the way the word is now used as an adjective: sickly sweet with a bitter, chemical aftertaste.

Equal, the most well-known sweetener, contains the less bitter-tasting aspartame, which is derived from the amino acids L-aspartic acid and L-phenylalanine. On cafe tables and in diet foods since 1981, aspartame contains 24 calories (100 kJ) per teaspoon but because it's 180 times sweeter than sugar, a little goes a long way.

NutraSweet also contains aspartame, while **Hermesetas** uses a blend of aspartame and sweetening agent Acesulphame K.

Splenda gets its sweetness from sucralose, which has been around since 1998 and is found in ice-cream, sauces and jellies. It's made from real sugar and tastes the closest to the real deal. To create it, food scientists substitute chlorine atoms for three hydrogen-oxygen groups on the sucrose molecule. That makes Splenda a tongue tingling 600 times sweeter than sugar.

Stevia, a natural sweetener with no aspartame or saccharin, derived from the stevia plant has .6 calories per stick. This is the only sweetener I'd recommend.

Sweet spices such as cinnamon and nutmeg are also spectacular sugar replacements and flow well into a steaming cup of coffee.

High fructose corn syrup (HFCS) is the worst type of sweetener made from maize or corn that, thankfully, is not used much here in Australia. The body is not able to process it well and it creates high levels of the triglyceride fats. Manufacturers use it because it's cheaper; it is a common ingredient in soft drinks in the US, where concerns have been raised. Research and animal testing has shown evidence that it may increase the risk of metabolic syndrome, which is an umbrella term for a number of health problems such as insulin resistance, high blood pressure and obesity.

UNDERSTANDING SWEET PACKAGING

Ingredient lists will commonly use technical words that many of us don't understand: if the words 'partially hydrogenated' or 'shortening' appear anywhere then the product contains trans fat. Stay away from foods that have anything more than 4 grams of sugar per serving (unless it's pure fruit). Any words that end with 'ose' or 'ol' are bad news: dextrose and sucrose mean sugar, and ingredients such as mannitol are alcohols that are quickly converted to sugar.

While we know all about fats, food labellers aren't required by law to include any information about fructose, so labels only say 'sugar' and lump them all together. Luckily weightloss warriors come with a built-in fructose detector—our tongues! If it tastes sweet, it probably contains fructose. If you're trying to lose weight, 50 grams a day is all that's recommended .

NinjaNewsflash
DRUNK ON SUGAR
Nearly all drinks are sweetened with sugar and therefore fructose. Drinking fructose in the form of fruit juices and soft drinks is dangerous because you can ingest large quantities of fructose with no other elements (such as fibre, carbohydrates, proteins or fat) to trigger your appetite control. If you're thirsty, drink water. Soft drinks are almost 6 per cent fructose by weight. This translates to 10 grams of body fat for the average 375 ml can of soft drink. Fruit juices are worse than soft drinks at 7 per cent fructose by weight. Sugary drinks are sweet poison.

To come down from a sugar high, you have to know how much you're hitting up in the first place. So take note of fake sugars and sugars in disguise by reading labels. Current Aussie guidelines (which haven't been revised in 30 years) recommend only 10–12 per cent of your daily energy intake should come from sugar—that's around 12 teaspoons for chicks.

Which is not to say you should join the Fake Sugar Tribe. About 66 per cent of Aussies are sweet on artificial sweeteners, with around 51 per cent consuming them via diet soft drinks or energy drinks. But while the three biggies—saccharin, aspartame and sucralose—hardly contain any calories, one glance at Australia's collective flab makes you wonder ... sugar replacements certainly don't seem to be helping us lose weight.

Artificial sweeteners are actually worse for you than table sugar. They act like stomach teasers: as you gulp Diet Coke your body anticipates the arrival of calories, when those calories don't show, your body sends you looking elsewhere for them—in the fridge, pantry and packets.

Sweeteners have been marketed as an alternative to sugar for those who are diabetic or trying to lose weight, but only in moderation, as they actually intensify your sweet tooth. The variety of intense sweeteners available are actually *sweeter* than sugar, making foods and drinks taste sweet while providing no energy (calories). So when you do eat real sugar it doesn't taste sweet enough and you're forced to reach for Extra— or extra.

The wasted warrior

Alcohol is linked to weight gain and obesity, not only because it's high in calories but also because it lessens the body's ability to burn fat. Excess alcohol consumption or alcohol abuse has been linked to high blood pressure, heart and liver disease and even some types of cancer. A drinking binge can also drastically reduce the amount of testosterone in your body by increasing the amount of the muscle-wasting hormone cortisol. On top of this alcohol reduces our ability to make healthy choices, affecting our judgement and increasing our appetite. How often have you headed for a Macca's drive-through or grabbed a greasy kebab after a big night out? Alcohol can give you a hangover in more ways than one—like that muffin top hanging over your jeans!

The way our bodies deal with alcohol is similar to how they deal with excess carbs: when we overeat carbohydrates they replace the body's fat as a source of energy to burn. Only a small portion of the alcohol consumed is converted into fat; the liver converts most of it into acetate, which is then released into the bloodstream. It's the increased amount of acetate that replaces fat as a source of energy and hampers fat being burned as energy. To lose weight we need to burn off excess fat and use it as fuel for our bodies—so anything that gets in the way of that will steer us off our weightloss warrior path.

Adding sugar to alcohol—like in cocktails—makes it even worse! Alcohol inhibits fat burning while your body works hard to eliminate the toxins from your liver. One night of binge drinking followed by high-fat, high-carb indulgences will ruin all your hard work and quickly set you back. Not to mention the fact that weightloss warriors need to have their sleep (alcohol decreases your REM sleep and even one glass robs you of a deep sleep cycle) and all their senses about them if they're to progress to black belt status!

Tiff's Tip

Ban the premix can! One UDL Vodka Green Apple has 230 calories (963 kJ), one Lemon Ruski has 220 calories (920 kJ) and one can of Bundy Rum and Cola has a whopping 275 calories (1,151 kJ).

BEST OF A BAD BUNCH

Swap 450 ml of beer (170 calories (711 kJ)) for 450 ml of light beer (125 calories (523 kJ))

Swap 30 ml scotch with 125 ml Coke (120 calories (502 kJ)) for 30 ml scotch and soda (70 calories (293 kJ))

Swap Mai Tai cocktail (235 calories (983 kJ)) for Margarita (110 calories (460 kJ))

Swap 100 ml glass of white wine (75 calories (313 kJ)) for wine spritzer (white wine with soda) (20 calories (83 kJ))

Better still, be like me and abstain altogether!

NinjaMove
MIX IT UP
Mix your drink with soda water to lower calories or drink a glass of water in between. Try a Cosmopolitan mocktail with cranberry juice and a twist of lime, or a Virgin Mary—tomato juice with pepper or Tabasco.

Expresso yourself

Add one latte a day to your diet without increasing your exercise and you'll add 7 kilos in one year. Coffee can be FULL of calories! It's easy to visit Starbucks and get a grande with extra cream, syrups and sweeteners and gulp down 500-plus calories (2,093 kJ). Some coffee concoctions equate to eating a meal.

Coca-Cola is basically made up of a cocktail of carbonated water, sugar, caffeine, phosphoric acid, colour and flavourings. One can (355 ml) contains 39 grams of carbohydrates, all of which come from 10 teaspoons worth of sugar. It's high in calories and simple carbohydrates (which when consumed excessively can lead to weight gain) as well as sugar and acid (which can cause the erosion of tooth enamel and tooth decay). Coke also contains high levels of phosphate, which is suspected of lowering the body's calcium levels and is not good news for kids as it can mean more broken bones due to poor bone mineralisation. High levels of phosphates in the blood basically pulls calcium off the bones, which can lead to serious conditions such as osteoporosis in adults.

COFFEE CALORIES (PER 300 ML CUP, WITH FULL-FAT MILK)

Macchiato (80 ml): 15 calories (62 kJ); 1 gram fat

Cafe mocha: 240 calories (1,004 kJ); 10 grams fat

Flat white: 170 calories (711 kJ); 10 grams fat

Caramel latte: 245 calories (1,025 kJ); 9 grams fat

Cafe latte: 170 calories (711 kJ); 10 grams fat

Chai latte: 260 calories (1,088 kJ); 8 grams fat

Cappuccino: 170 calories (711 kJ); 10 grams fat

Hot chocolate: 315 calories (1,318 kJ); 11 grams fat

Starbucks grande Java chip with whipped cream: 415 calories (1,737 kJ); 16 grams of fat

Hot chocolate with whipped cream: 555 calories (2,323 kJ)! 33 grams of fat!!

FIZZY CAFFEINE (PER 250 ML GLASS)

Coca-Cola = 48.75 mg caffeine

Pepsi Max = 44 mg caffeine

Diet Coke = 48 mg caffeine

Pepsi = 40 mg caffeine

Diet Pepsi = 44 mg caffeine

Diet Coke Caffeine-Free = 2 mg caffeine

NinjaNewsflash

DO YOU WANT FERTILISER WITH THAT?
What do hamburgers and fertiliser have in common? Turns out hamburgers, especially those served at fast food restaurants, are routinely treated with ammonia to kill off E. coli bacteria. That's the same substance used in fertilisers and household cleaners. Yum!

Tiff's Tip

Sugar is added to heaps of foods that don't need it, from the sesame bun in a McDonald's hamburger, to a Thai stir-fry ... not to mention those 27 grams of sugar in a bottle of vitamin water.

H₂*whoa!*

Your greatest weightloss warrior weapon is the most popular product on the market. It suppresses appetite, improves strength, increases speed, helps you lose stubborn fat, improves your complexion, keeps you alert, beats tiredness and helps you sleep well. It's your armour and your ammunition in the battle for good health and you'll never conquer the scales without it—and it's *free!*

Guessed yet? Yup, it's good old water.

Have you ever woken up in the morning and felt so groggy it was like having a hangover? If so, you were probably dehydrated. In fact a hangover—headache, tiredness and fatigue—is partially dehydration caused by the diuretic effects of alcohol. The days when we have trouble exercising, or can't get started, could easily be due to dehydration.

Dehydration decreases endurance, strength and physical performance. As you become dehydrated your body's core temperature increases, which affects your cardiovascular function and reduces your capacity for physical work. Even a small lowering of your body's hydration level, like 3 per cent of body weight, can decrease contractile strength by as much as 10 per cent!

Why we need water to lose fat

Water is the most abundant nutrient in your body: you are 70 per cent water. Even your bones are 20 per cent water. Water regulates your temperature, transports nutrients and builds tissue. If you don't water a plant, it dies; if you don't water yourself, you won't grow to your full potential. You can live for up to a month without food, but you'll die by the end of the week if you stop drinking water.

Every physiological process in your body depends on water, so dehydration has devastating effects if you're trying to burn fat. The restoration and rebalancing of your hormones occurs in water: when it comes time for your kidneys to eliminate toxic waste products and there isn't enough water to transfer the waste through urine, your body panics and instinctively retains water to survive. So dehydration, paradoxically, causes fluid retention. When water retention hits waste products can't be flushed out and pile up in your system, meaning your kidneys can't burn fat as efficiently as they should. The liver tries to help out with the overload but, while covering the kidneys, it gets behind on its own work.

Many people avoid drinking a lot of water because they think it will make them bloated, but the opposite is true: when you're dehydrated your body senses the lack of adequate water and holds on to what's currently in the body. When you consume adequate amounts of water your body senses that you're no longer dehydrated and your kidneys flush it all out of your system.

NinjaNewsflash
DON'T DRINK YOUR DAY AWAY
Juice, sports drinks and energy drinks—not to mention milk drinks and smoothies—'cost' more calories than you might think. Some sports drinks are nothing but sugar water, making up a quarter of your daily caloric intake and putting on more than you've just worked off! Not to mention the sodium!

Tiff's Tip

By the time you're experiencing the symptoms of a dry mouth, headache and lethargy, you've already lost a whole litre of water!

Tiff's Tip

If you only change one habit, increasing your water intake will have dramatic effects on your physique immediately.

But drinking more water means just that: not more coffee (dehydrating) or soft drinks (liquid lollies) or energy drinks (devil doses). Drinking ordinary water can fill you up without adding calories or sugar to your diet. Drinking just two 235 ml glasses of water before each meal can help you consume between 75–90 fewer calories (313 kJ–376 kJ) per meal. While artificially flavoured water and protein shakes may look fancier, it's ordinary tap water that will really help you lose weight. Spruce it up by spiking it with lemon, lime or cucumber slices to help your body absorb it more easily.

It's more likely to be sodium that's to blame for your bloating, not water. Excess sodium can raise your blood pressure and slow down your metabolism. It gets stored just beneath the skin where it attracts water that's retained in your cells, which makes you look puffy. And it's hidden in most products, especially packaged foods, frozen foods, canned foods and—the enemy of all weightloss warriors—fast foods. Oh, and condiments. Aussies love their tomato sauce, much to my English grandmother's disgust, who's seen us squirt it on everything, even lamb. A squeeze of tomato, sweet chilli or soy sauce could load you up with all the sodium you need for an entire day. To maximise your body's fat burning potential, I recommend no more than 6 grams of salt per day.

So get ya ninja on and get that water in!

Hey, Bad Blender!

Juice bars are bad news. Juicing converts fruit and vegetables from a food source containing significant fibre mass to one containing little other than fructose and water. Take a glass of 100 per cent fat-free apple: 14 grams fructose, 6 grams glucose and 4 grams sucrose, which is broken into its component fructose and glucose by our bodies adding 2 grams each to the totals of fructose and glucose. The now 8 grams glucose is 'counted' by our pancreas but the 16 grams of fructose is completely unseen and converted directly to about 7 grams of circulating fatty acid (4 calories (16 kJ) per gram of carbohydrate, 9 calories (37 kJ) per gram of fat).

Of the 96 calories (401 kJ) in my glass of apple juice, the appetite centre in my brain only sees the 32 calories (133 kJ) provided by the glucose. Sixty-four calories (267 kJ) slip through completely undetected while the fatty acids created from fructose in the bloodstream dull the effect of insulin, which means we have to make more insulin to respond to the calories we're detecting. Over time we become more and more insulin resistant: we eat more without feeling full. How sneaky!

And if you suffer from a sensitive stomach and regular bloating like me, fructose may be why.

Opt for fatty nutty smoothies with rice milk, LSA mix, crushed almonds and bananas over fruit juices. And remember, that's a meal, so add it to your daily calorie intake. Watch out for meal replacement shakes though—they have no thermic effect on your metabolism, and can count as more than one meal in your daily calorie intake, and rob you of the pleasure-fest of chewing. Worst of all, meal replacements teach you nothing about nutrition in life or battling the bulge.

NinjaMove

WATER IT IN

Higher protein diets do have a diuretic effect and require extra attention to water intake as the processing of protein foods generates metabolic waste products that have to be flushed out and removed by the kidneys. But it's a myth that high-protein diets cause kidney damage: a high protein diet isn't harmful to healthy kidneys as long as plenty of water is consumed.

NinjaNewsflash

Aussies consume the equivalent of 45 kilos of packaged sugar, per person, every year!

Tiff's Tip

Binge on diuretic vegies—
spinach, lettuce, all leafy
greens, dandelion, parsley,
asparagus and cucumber—to
get the best fat flush.

BUSTING LIQUID MYTHS

Drink more than eight glasses a day

Eight to ten glasses is a good start for a daily water intake, but if you're active—and weightloss warriors *are*—we should be talking litres not glasses. It's important to measure your water intake: try drinking out of the same bottle so you know whether you're really hydrated or not. Your skin, energy and bodily functions will all improve within days of drinking more water.

Drink before you're thirsty

Sedentary people might do fine drinking when they are thirsty but exercise blunts your thirst mechanism. You lose fluid so rapidly the brain can't respond in time. And women lose even more water exercising than men. Thirst is never a good indication of your level of hydration. An hour before you hit the gym, gulp an extra 600 ml so you can hydrate before you dehydrate—it takes 60 minutes for the liquid to travel from your gut to your muscles.

Tea and coffee don't only dehydrate you

Down two long blacks and you'll visit the ladies' room often enough to earn a VIP pass, but, despite its speedy exit, the liquid in your favourite morning caffeine boost still counts towards your hydration goal. After all, it's *mostly* water. The key to consuming caffeinated beverages is moderation: too many will dehydrate and disrupt your hormonal balance.

Bottled isn't necessarily better

Unless you're travelling, what comes from the tap is as nutritious as water gets. Aussie tap water contains minerals like sodium, calcium, magnesium and zinc. Purified and distilled waters are boiled during processing to strip them of any trace minerals. Shop-bought H_2O also lacks the fluoride that comes with our water supply. Plus you're hurting the planet every time you buy another bottle—Australia's current annual consumption of bottled water generates more than 60,000 tonnes of greenhouse gas emissions! Not to mention the money you're throwing away: one litre of bottled water is up to 2500 times the cost of tap water.

Energy drinks exposed

Energy drinks are designed to increase stamina, mental alertness and performance and usually contain high amounts of caffeine, taurine and glucuronoactone. And, often, sugar. Taurine and glucuronoactone occur naturally in the body, but their effects—when consumed in the high doses in which they appear in energy drinks—are still being studied. We already know that excessive amounts of caffeine can have an effect on developing brains, as well as negative effects on the immune system. Consuming two or more cans of energy drinks per day can lead to sleep problems, anxiety, irritability and bed wetting in children. Even the manufacturers warn not to exceed two to five cans a day and advise that people who are sensitive to caffeine or suffering from heart problems should be careful. I say we all should be.

NinjaMove

FINDING WATER IN FOODS
To help cut calories, eat water-rich foods like vegetables: the water travels through the stomach and into the intestines along with the rest of the meal, making you feel full without adding to the meal's calorie count. Drinking water satisfies your thirst but eating foods high in water satiates hunger and hydrates you as well. Choose broth-based soups like chicken noodle, or fresh juicy fruits and vegies like watermelon, cucumber and tomato.

NinjaNewsflash

GIVE YOURSELF A SPORTING CHANCE
So-called 'sports' drinks are jammed full of sugar—up to 40 grams. That's equivalent to eating 150 grams of M&M's or 2 cups of chocolate ice-cream. Powerade has 280 calories (1,172 kJ), 220 mg of sodium and 76 grams of sugar! Like Gatorade it's made by Coke for elite athletes like Lance Armstrong who need dramatic replenishment after gruelling exercise. The problem is it's marketed to everyone. If you're exercising super hard and need to replenish electrolytes take Gastrolyte or add two capfuls of Gatorade to a glass of water.

'*Biggest Loser* contestants anticipated being told they had to eat less food, but were shocked when they found out it was the kinds of foods they were eating that had to change if they were to lose weight.'

DEADLY DOZEN—THE TWELVE WORST FOODS

Ice-cream, soft cheeses—instead opt for full-fat Greek yoghurt or non-milk fruit sorbet, cottage cheese, ricotta cheese, low-fat hard cheeses, rice milk, fetta cheese, goat's milk.

Fried foods—choose grilled, steamed or ideally raw foods.

Doughnuts and pastries—just get ya ninja on and go cold turkey!

Chocolate and lollies—try berries or a few squares of dark or sugar-free chocolate.

Soft drinks—opt for soda/mineral water with lime or lemon—or just good old-fashion, fat-blasting tap water!

Fruit drinks/sweetened drinks—switch to freshly made vegie juices with ginger, lemon or mint.

Alcohol—try low-calorie, low-carb, low-alcohol beverages.

Processed meats—opt for lean, organic meats or fresh meats cut 'off the bone'.

White bread, canned pasta in sauce, lasagne sheets—choose sourdough/spelt bread, vermicelli or rice pasta; try wholemeal mountain bread instead of lasagne sheets.

All fast foods! All naked foods!

Biscuits and chips—choose unsalted nuts, unbuttered popcorn, Vita-Weats, rice or corn cakes, muesli bars (watch the sugar, though), organic natural yoghurt.

Sugary breakfast cereals—switch to oats, muesli with fresh berries, homemade muesli.

Tiff's Tip

Try a cup of aloe vera juice for a shot of vitamins and minerals. Made from organically grown aloe plants it works as an inner gel to support and maintain a healthy digestive system.

Secret agents

Chew **parsley** for fresh breath. Parsley combats bacteria that causes bad breath and plaque. It's also a natural diuretic so will fight bloating and puffiness.

Cop the **copper** in cashews, walnuts, shellfish, whole grains, olives and—here's the good news—chocolate! Copper aids melanin production, the pigment that gives hair its colour, so low levels can lead to premature greying.

Try **soba**. If you have a sensitive stomach like me, swap to soba noodles. They contain about 20 per cent less wheat, which is what brings about the bloat.

Embrace the **brazil nut**, an awesome source of omega-3 fatty acids, which can increase the sheen on your hair.

Be sure to have **healthy fats** at every meal as many nutrients are fat-soluble (and therefore better absorbed when eaten with a healthy fat).

Try **sautéing**, grilling, baking or just blanching vegies as the **water-soluble nutrients** easily get lost in the cooking process. Microwaving broccoli preserves 90 per cent of the vitamin C versus 66 per cent with boiling or steaming.

Heat **tomatoes**! Tomatoes contain lycopene, a potent antioxidant that combats aging, stroke and heart disease. Cooking tomatoes or using tomato paste can increase bioavailability of lycopene by up to 500 per cent.

NinjaMove

AVOID THE BREAKFAST FAT BOMB
The iced cinnamon roll is one of the worst cellulite feeders with 5 grams of trans fat, 390 calories (1,632 kJ), 20 grams sugar and 19 grams of saturated fat. Never start your day with a bloated ball of bad fats and sugar!

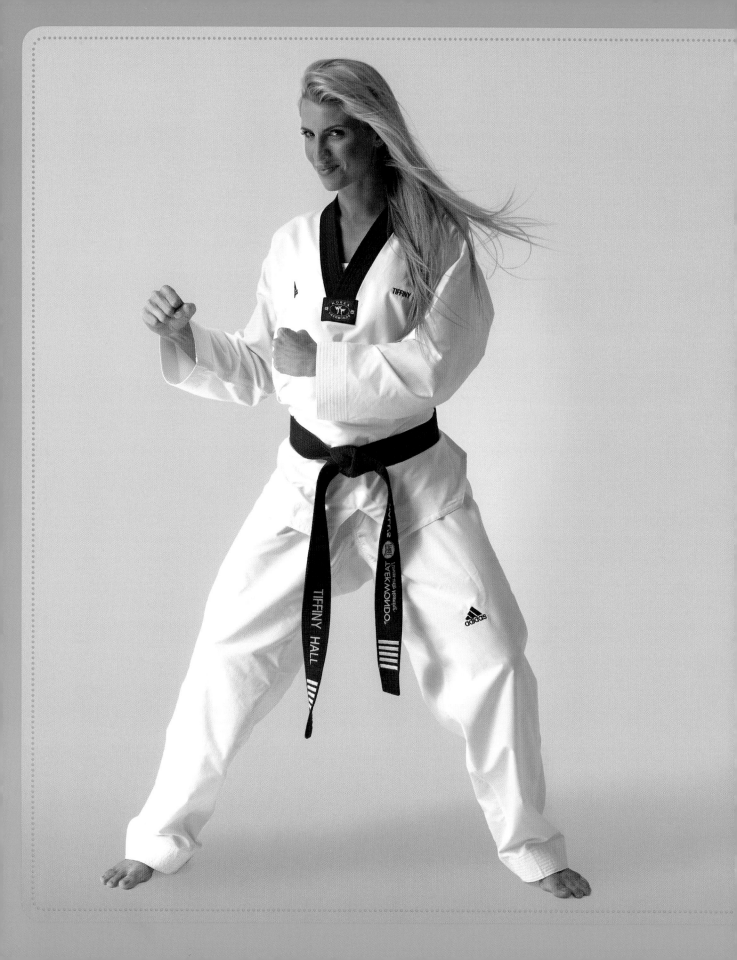

Blue belt: Warrior vitality

'SPEED UP YOUR METABOLISM BY HARMONISING
YOUR HORMONES. EXERCISE IS YOUR WEAPON
OF MASS REDUCTION!'

You're already fighting

You probably don't know it, or haven't thought about it, but you already have a fat-fighting ninja on your side. It's your metabolism. Every time you eat, enzymes in your cells break down the food and turn it into energy that keeps your neurons firing, your heart beating and your legs pumping.

Your metabolism is like a furnace—the more fuel you put on the fire, the stronger, faster and longer it burns. Weightloss warriors need a well-stoked furnace. My greatest asset is my well-trained metabolism: it keeps me on the warrior path even if I slip up with my taekwondo training, or don't eat naked for a few days. You can burn up to an extra 600 calories (2,511 kJ) a day just by eating more often. This is called raising your 'resting metabolic rate' or RMR (the amount of calories you burn while at rest).

Metabolism is often described as an engine, which weight-loss products claim to be able to kick-start, speed up or rev. But it's really more like a chemistry lab—a delicate reaction in which molecules, hormones and cell messenger chemicals control how quickly you burn calories.

All bodily functions are controlled by your hormones. Whenever you eat, your body's glands release hormones to help you balance your blood sugar, go to sleep, burn fat or build muscle. How much of each hormone is released depends on the type of calories you ate, when you ate them, how much you ate and whether you exercised.

Most weight-loss 'miracle cures' only work on one hormone at a time, but to win the fat fight once and for all warriors must ensure their arsenal of hormones and glands are all working harmoniously. To do this, our Weapons of Mass Digestion are KNOWLEDGE and nude foods. To rebalance our metabolism, we need to first understand our hormones.

The hormonal (or endocrine) system comprises glands that secrete hormones, the hormones themselves, the way they act on the body, and the way they interact with each other. Complicated, huh? Bear with me. Hormones are the body's chemical messengers—couriers, if you like, that zoom through the bloodstream, delivering messages to our body's organs and tissues.

These hormones are pumped out by different glands in your body, one of which is your thyroid. It's a butterfly-shaped gland just below your Adam's apple that controls the amount of oxygen each cell uses, the rate at which your body burns calories, overall growth, digestion, body temperature and even mood. The hormones produced by the thyroid can speed up or slow down your metabolism. If you starve yourself the thyroid becomes sluggish. When your thyroid's out of whack, chemical reactions all over the body cause a heap of problems. If it's going too fast or too slow that affects your energy levels and weight. So does the balance of the other hormones in your body.

All the hormones work together to fan your metabolic fire, but there are some that are more crucial to hunger than others—insulin, leptin and ghrelin. Sex and stress hormones also affect your hunger.

NinjaMove

LATE-NIGHT LOCKOUT

I know the evening's supposed to be romantic but eating in the dark is dangerous—and not because you might stab yourself in the eye with a fork! Night-time calories hang around, day-time ones can be used in running around, so close the kitchen at 9 pm and you should shut out some unwanted fat too.

Insulin

You've probably heard of this one—it's the hormone that's involved in diabetes. Insulin is produced in the pancreas, an organ perched behind your stomach. The pancreas plays a critical role in how the body reacts to food. Within minutes of a meal your pancreas pumps out a series of insulin surges. Insulin's main gig is to lower your blood sugar by either ushering sugar into the liver to convert it to glucose for muscles to use, or shuttling fatty acids into fat cells. Lower insulin levels help your body burn stored fat for fuel.

Insulin has to work to keep your weight in check. For example, if you eat a Tim Tam on an empty stomach your blood sugar surges, insulin overreacts and works twice as hard as normal to cleanse the sugar from your blood. The overworking insulin doesn't leave enough glucose circulating in your bloodstream so your blood sugar crashes, kicking off the starving/stuffing cycle. This is the root of sugar addiction. When the muscles are already full of sugar where do the extra calories go? Straight to fat. When excess insulin lurks in your bloodstream your body can't tap into your fat stores.

If you starve-then-stuff often enough your pancreas produces more insulin, which your cells will eventually start to ignore. Shut out from your muscle factories the sugar is abandoned to roam about your blood. Hello, type 2 diabetes!

Leptin

While the boffins keep discovering new hormones, this one we know really well. Leptin is produced in fat cells and works with our thyroid gland and other hormones to help our bodies regulate hunger. Leptin is most active in your brain. When you eat, fat cells all over your body release leptin that then travels to your brain to regulate appetite. Leptin switches on appetite-suppressing signals and also helps the body to tap into longer-term fat stores. When leptin isn't working you're no longer a weightloss warrior, but a warrior on a warpath of food destruction.

Usually having too little leptin is not a problem as the more fat you have, the more leptin you produce. But when the body continually cranks out excess levels of leptin in response to overeating the receptors for leptin can start to wear out and no longer recognise the hormone. If you lose a few kilos your body will become more sensitive to leptin and it will help you stop eating when you're full.

Tiff's Tip

Remember:
Eat every 4 hours. Just eating and digesting can make up 10 per cent of your body's metabolic rate—keeping leptin and ghrelin under control.

Ghrelin

Ghrelin acts as the Yin to leptin's Yang—they work in harmony to balance hunger and fullness (also called satiety). Just as leptin tells the brain to turn off hunger, ghrelin tells the brain you're starving. Produced in the guts when you're hungry, or about to eat, or even just thinking about something yummy, your gut releases ghrelin. Ghrelin then trots off to your brain to turn your appetite-control knob up and your calorie-burning knob down.

Ghrelin rises when your stomach's empty. That's why you feel hungry at certain times of the day, because your body clock relies on ghrelin to remind you to eat. Since it takes ghrelin a few minutes to tell your brain you're full eating slowly can help you to eat less.

As it rises, ghrelin helps you sleep and allows the release of Human Growth Hormone (HGH). Your hunger hormone needs to be high-ish when you go to bed so you can slip into deep sleep. Carbs depress ghrelin faster than any other nutrient, so eating carbs before bed is definitely not a warrior habit. When you sleep, you want to reach stage 4 sleep, because that's when a big hit of HGH comes to help protect leptin levels. Don't go to bed starving, just not full.

Ghrelin is a clever gremlin in getting you to eat—it even triggers reward centres in the brain to make food look better than it is. For some people, passing a bakery displaying hot, fresh doughnuts can be the same as an addict shooting up. Constant dieting keeps ghrelin levels high, which is why you can feel hungrier when on a diet. It's hardly fair.

Human Growth Hormone

HGH has a black belt in everything—it builds muscle, burns fat, keeps your heart healthy, protects bones, aids overall health and even makes you happier. It also plays a big part in the growth of bone and body tissue and is ace for the immune system. HGH stops muscle breaking down, which keeps your resting metabolic rate up and enables you to power your exercise. HGH also helps to tap in to your fat stores because fat cells have growth hormone receptors that trigger your cells to break down and burn, baby, BURN. This hormone also discourages your fat cells from absorbing or holding on to any fat floating around your bloodstream—that's the kind of ninja we want on our side!

During intense exercise HGH shuns glucose and instead encourages the body to use fat as fuel. HGH is one of the most important reasons to exercise. Sleeping well, chilling out more and eliminating environmental toxins will also help you to rebalance your HGH level.

Tiff's Tip

Find people who are with you on your warrior path. Avoid the 'It's too hard' haters or the 'Maybe one day' dreamers. Challenge yourself to stand out and, with time, you may become a leader for others to follow.

Oestrogen

Oestrogen isn't just a chick hormone that gives us boobs and periods. Guys have it too, in their testes and adrenals, helping them maintain healthy brain function and sex drive. In women these hormones are produced in our ovaries, fat tissues, adrenals, and in pregnancy, the placenta. Men and women produce oestrogen naturally but we also cop a dose from our environment and food. Oestrogen helps to regulate our moods and impacts on our blood fats, digestive enzymes, water and salt balance, bone density, heart function and memory. While it puts fat on our bums and hips, that fat helps our insulin response. Most importantly for weightloss warriors it helps to regulate our appetites.

As you head towards menopause your body shuts down production of this chemical, which shifts the fat from your hips and booty to your belly. This belly oestrogen is called oestrone. If you stop exercising, you hold more fat around your stomach; the more fat you have, the more oestrone you'll produce. I know, unfair again, right? It's a vicious cycle because more insulin means more oestrone and more oestrone means more stomach fat; and more stomach fat means still more oestrone.

Testosterone

And this one is not just for guys. Don't worry ladies; boosting these hormones won't make us look like Arnie. Instead think libido, energy, motivation, and building lean sexy muscle to churn calories. Remember, the more lean muscle mass you have, the greater your power to burn up a burger just by sleeping!

Testosterone is an anabolic hormone: it builds rather than breaks down muscle. A force for good in the metabolic fight. We reduce production of it as we age, but exercise at any age, good fats and proteins as well as adequate zinc and vitamin B, boost testosterone.

Cortisol

Cortisol is our fight-or-flight hormone and gets us out of some pretty ugly situations. But though the heart-pumping effects soon pass cortisol's fat-storing legacy hangs around. Our adrenal glands pump out cortisol in all kinds of stressful situations: when you run to catch a train; lunge to stop your kid darting into traffic; or miss a step on the stairs.

Everyone gets stressed, and you can't get rid of all stress. Trying to lose weight can be very stressful. The problem with constant stress is that it shuts down our fat burn. When you first get stressed norepinephrine tells your body to stop producing insulin so that you have plenty of fast-acting blood sugar on hand to run, act fast, or freak out.

Epinephrine will relax the muscles of the stomach and intestines and decrease blood flow to these organs—since your body would rather save your life than digest your food. Once stress passes and digestion resumes cortisol continues to have a big impact on weight loss, particularly on how your body uses fuel.

Tiff's Tip

Go green! Green tea gives a caffeine boost but also promotes fat burning and improves insulin sensitivity. Aim for 2-3 cups a day.

WARRIOR BODY AWARENESS: WHAT HAPPENS …

When you cry
Crying is a release. A cleanse. An emotional detox. The act of crying releases hormones and chemicals from your body. Scientists have discovered that emotional tears contain high levels of manganese and a chemical called prolactin. It's believed that crying is a way of removing excess chemicals that aren't good for the body, which may explain why we tend to feel better after having a cry. Your heart rate increases but afterwards when your breathing returns to normal you'll be infused with a feeling of calm. The longer you cry the happier you'll feel afterwards, as it takes longer for your body to return to a normal rate of breathing than it did for you to get upset. The period of deep breathing reduces stress levels.

When you smoke
The moment you inhale you begin doing damage to your body. A mixture of gases is instantly released around your eyes, nose and throat. The cilia, which help to keep the bronchial tubes and lungs clean, are momentarily paralysed. When you cough, they have come back to life. When you inhale, the carbon monoxide robs the muscles, brain and blood of oxygen, making the whole body, especially the heart, work harder. The tar coats the lungs, which can cause lung and throat cancer. Over a year a pack-a-day smoker will ingest a full cup of tar. Smoking does not relieve stress: the feeling of relaxation that smokers experience is actually a return to the normal state non-smokers experience all the time.

When you kiss
Kissing releases the hormone oxytocin, which encourages you to bond and lowers levels of cortisol. Receiving another person's germs also helps to boost the immune system. Lots of things happen to the body when you kiss. Hormones are released and adrenalin rises causing your blood pressure to increase and warm the body. Your heart beat increases to about 60–100 beats a minute. As adrenalin levels increase, serotonin (the body's feel-good chemical) actually decreases, keeping us focused and more impulsive. The neurotransmitter dopamine is also released into the brain causing pleasure and making you want more. That's a lot going on!

When you laugh
A deep belly laugh produces feel-good chemicals such as endorphins and dopamine. These help ward off depression and provide pleasure. Even if you don't feel like laughing, smile. Your brain will mirror your emotions. Laughing bubbles you up. It boosts your immune system, decreases stress hormones and increases immune cells and infection-fighting antibodies.

When you eat chocolate
Chocolate in moderation triggers the yeah-baby! chemicals in your brain that make you feel happier immediately. The occasional piece of dark chocolate benefits our circulatory system by reducing blood pressure, is rich in antioxidants and can help to lower cholesterol levels.

When you run
Your body temperature increases, encouraging your blood to move more quickly. Your body then begins to use your carbohydrate stores to fuel these actions. After 10 minutes your body finds a zone where you're running on autopilot. Running will boost your endorphins and make you feel awesome—as good as a line of chocolate.

Cortisol tells your body what fat, protein or carbohydrates to burn and when to burn them depending on what kind of challenge you face. When the body needs more energy cortisol can either move fat to the muscles for burning or break down muscle and convert it to glycogen. While cortisol suppresses appetite initially—who wants to eat when they're about to be punched in the face?!—any leftover cortisol increases your cravings. That's why when you're close to deadline the grilled vegie salad just won't cut it.

Then, once you eat, your body releases a cascade of rewarding brain chemicals that help you to feel 'de-stressed'. Your clever brain chemicals anchor happy to feeling full and can trigger that binge-eating addiction every time your boyfriend doesn't text you back. You feel better once you eat and eventually you become physically and psychologically dependent on that release to manage stress. The reality is you don't need chocolate; you need to chill out.

Food shouldn't be a stress management tool. Self-medicating with food will only increase cortisol in your body. When stress continues over time your body resists weight loss because it doesn't want to add starving to its stressful list of things to do, so it hoards food and fat, turning young fat cells into mature fat cells that stick with us forever. Great.

Some lucky people may have mellow adrenal reactions to stressful situations, but many of us tend to overreact because we've trained our stress response system—like we've trained our metabolism, our muscles, and our thought patterns. We've become addicted to stress.

Hormonal imbalance

A hormonal imbalance occurs when there's too much or too little of a particular hormone, causing the body's systems to function abnormally. Being overweight is the most common cause of hormonal imbalance. (Other causes include birth-control pills and devices, genetics, stress, lack of exercise and tumours.) If a hormone imbalance is left untreated it can lead to serious health concerns, such as thyroid problems, metabolic syndrome, chronic Premenstrual Syndrome (PMS), Premenstrual Dysphoric Disorder (PMDD) and even diabetes. Weightloss warriors need to retrain their bodies to restore natural balance and metabolic harmony. (And please, if you have serious symptoms, see your GP.)

NinjaMove

WRITE IT OUT

When I can't get to sleep 'cause my mind's buzzing, I take a big fat texta and write down everything I'm stressed about. By taking it out of the thinking world and into the doing world, I can sleep easy knowing I'll find a solution when the sun rises.

Helping your hormones

High-fibre foods—the more fibre the better our natural oestrogen system works. It also keeps the ghrelin gremlins happy. Found in bran, oatmeal, peas, strawberries, wholemeal breads, cabbage, carrots and cauliflower.

High-protein foods—improve leptin sensitivity, which results in lower calorie uptake. Up your protein intake to 30 per cent of each meal.

Vitamin C—helps reduce cortisol levels. All fruits and vegies contain the big C. Cantaloupe, capsicums, tomatoes, broccoli and sweet potatoes are my favourite.

Allicin—found in garlic and onions, helps boost testosterone and inhibits cortisol, which can compete with testosterone.

Niacin—helps boost testosterone levels. Found in dairy products, lean meats, nuts and eggs.

Zinc—also boots testosterone levels. Hit up oysters, beef, turkey, yoghurt, cheddar cheese, cashews, baked beans.

Big breakfasts—keep ghrelin from grumbling. I'm thinking a vegetarian eggwhite omelette, bowl of oats and berries, or half a sliced banana and a small yoghurt—not a brekkie burrito the size of your head with sour cream and bacon!

Eating to a schedule—pack a sachet of almonds in your bag or take tabouleh to your desk to keep the hunger hormones at bay.

Green vegies—any foods with high water content count as high-volume and keep ghrelin levels low.

All omega-3—these good fatties kickstart your metabolism and raise leptin levels if your fat furnace has slowed down. Dig in to fatty fish like salmon, as well as walnuts, olive oil and flaxseeds.

Hindering your hormones

A massive dinner—delays leptin release until 2 hours after the meal!

Alcohol—drinking too much makes you a munching monster, increases oestrogen, decreases testosterone, raises cortisol … you know the drill.

Caffeine—affects most hormones, so keep it under control.

Invisible fat (sugar, especially fructose)—affects leptin and ghrelin.

Processed carbs—these and fat foes block leptin and ghrelin and increase oestrogen levels.

Bakery walk-by—gets ghrelin going. Don't cave to the crave.

Eating in the dark—affects ghrelin and insulin.

Licorice—interferes with cortisol and testosterone. I know, I'm crying: chocolate bullets are my all-time favourite. Just indulge occasionally and you'll be fine.

Manufactured 'low-fat' 'low-protein' foods—mess with ghrelin and testosterone.

Gluten—can cause elevated cortisol levels if you are intolerant. Many people are gluten-intolerant and don't know it. If you're concerned, try gluten-free products or just cut down on wheat products.

Tiff's Tip

Us ladies are supposed to have a bit of fat on our hips and butt—that's where the hormone good guys leptin and adiponectin hang out. But watch that muffin top, which is toxic visceral fat.

Sleeping (and your hormones)

Sleep is so important for health. Sleep chemically rebalances your brain. Deep sleep regulates your metabolism. In fact, an hour after we go to sleep we release our greatest pulse of growth hormone, the hormone that prompts the body to burn stored fat. So fat burns while you sleep as well as when you exercise, just as muscles rebuild and grow when you rest. So sleep is obviously integral to weight loss.

Sleep energises you for exercise, and exercise is a great way to reset your clock in the mornings. Activity increases oxygen in the blood to wake you up and stop you from reaching for the snooze button—or a sugary coffee and cinnamon scroll on the way to work. Our appetite-control hormones and the rest of our metabolism is directly affected by how much sleep we get. Have you ever experienced a sleepless night followed by a day when, no matter what you eat, you never feel full or satisfied? That's because of leptin and ghrelin; together these hormones work in a kind of check-and-balance system to control feelings of hunger and fullness.

Two sleepless nights will cut your 'I'm full' hormone, leptin, by 20 per cent, as well as increasing your hunger by 30 per cent. This jab, then cross-punch, combination makes you much more likely to snack on high-carb treats.

Smoking (and your hormones)

We all know smoking is a major bummer for your entire body, but did you know exercise can help you kick the habit by releasing endorphins and reducing cravings? Many people keep smoking for fear of gaining weight—the best way to stop that is to exercise. Exercise delivers a double-knockout punch: it repairs your damaged lungs and helps you combat cravings. If you quit smoking you'll breathe easier and exercise more and the cancer stick will no longer appeal.

Alcohol (and your hormones)

Booze releases oestrogen into your bloodstream, promotes fat storage and decreases muscle growth. As soon as that first sip slides down, your body gobbles up all the glycogen in your liver, making you hungry and reducing your inhibitions so you don't think twice about scoffing the party pies. You also burn way less fat, and burn it more slowly.

If you like a tipple, stick to wine, especially organic wines, which are produced without pesticides or too many preservatives (which can give you that cheap wine hangover). You'll soon learn to taste the difference.

NinjaNewsflash

HORMONE TRAUMA

Three million Aussies have diabetes or pre-diabetes. Nearly a million Aussies have thyroid problems. One in three of us over 25 years old have metabolic syndrome. Don't become a statistic!

Tiff's Tip

Cut carbs just before bed. Your hunger hormone should be high as you slip into deep sleep—carbs depress ghrelin faster than any other nutrient, so eating carbs will delay your entry into deeper sleep for several hours.

Caffeine (and your hormones)

Pure caffeine in moderate doses (200–400 mg daily) can elevate metabolism by up to 6 per cent, improve cognitive function and even improve insulin sensitivity. The problem is that coffee often comes with cream, milk, sugar and syrups, which can make your cuppa equal to a whole meal's calories. Adding one extra full-fat milk latte to your day equates to a 7-kilo weight gain in 1 year!

Ever noticed how you crave the muffin between first and second cups of coffee? That's because excess caffeine stimulates the stress hormones. If you sip caffeinated drinks all day, switching from V to Red Bull to coffee to Coke, you're triggering stress in your body. Caffeinated drinks are also a diuretic, draining precious water from your body so you can't even flush out the toxins. When you're dehydrated your blood volume decreases, reducing the amount of oxygen that can get to your muscles. So enjoy your caffeine the way nature intended—organic coffee with minimal milk and sugar, and don't forget to hydrate with water.

NinjaNewsflash

WHY SHOULD YOU MOVE?
You'll live longer. You'll have stronger bones. You'll be more chilled. You'll be richer, with all the cash you save from being healthier! Life gets easier—you can carry groceries, do chores and wrestle the kids with warrior speed and grace.

PREPARE FOOD TO MINIMISE HORMONAL DAMAGE

Remove visible fat and skin from chicken, meat and fish.

Wash vegetable and fruit skins to eliminate pesticide residue—use gentle dish soap that doesn't contain scents or phosphates.

Remove outer layers of cabbage and lettuce.

Chop off the tops of fruits such as apples to avoid pesticides that might have drained into the area.

Wash reusable plastic drink bottles by hand, not in the dishwasher. Or better still use recyclable stainless steel bottles for water.

Grill, bake or poach meats. Avoid frying them.

Avoid Mystery Meats such as hot dogs, bologna sausage and frankfurt sausages.

Buy glass food storage containers instead of plastic ones.

Stay away from canned food as much as possible by eating seasonal produce.

Never microwave with plastic wrap, use a chlorine-free paper towel to cover a dish or invert another dish on top.

Don't buy boil-in-a-bag microwave rice or vegies.

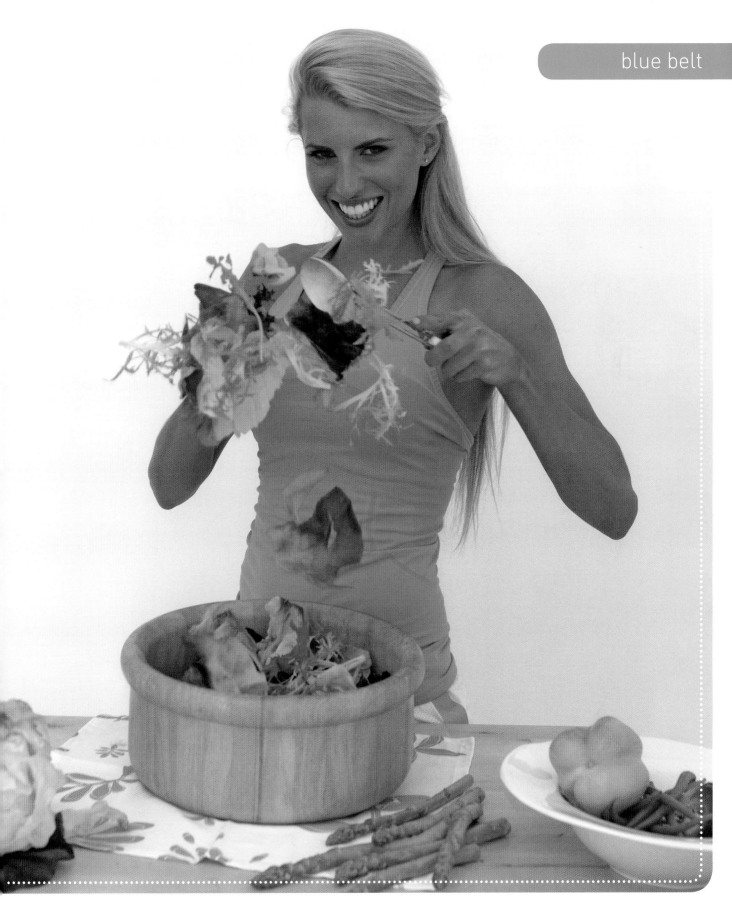

> **Tiff's Tip**
>
> What you eat determines
> the size of your body but it's
> exercise that determines
> its shape.

The ultra importance of exercise

Wanna know a ninja secret? Weightloss warriors aren't fooled by fad diets; they know exercise is the essential ingredient to achieving real, lasting health and happiness. Luckily your body has an elemental need to get physical, just as it needs oxygen, sleep and water. When you exercise, your body rewards you with endorphins—the 'feel good' chemicals that also combat stress. That's to keep you coming back for more.

Choose a form of cardio that you enjoy. You might like exercising outdoors, indoors, group fitness, bootcamps, sports or even a DVD in the living room while the kids are sleeping (and no, I don't mean a *Gossip Girl* DVD!)

When everything is in balance your body will be at peace. When your body's at peace, your mind can rest, and when your mind's at rest, your spirit will soar!

Each kilo of muscle burns three times—THREE TIMES!—as many calories as a kilo of fat. Muscles absorb blood sugar and enhance your body's insulin sensitivity.

To earn your blue belt in health, you have to move like the wind! When you train hard, the fat-burning growth hormone is released, which reduces cortisol, boosts testosterone and makes cells more sensitive to insulin. Exercising intensely, even if for only brief periods, increases your metabolism-boosting thyroid hormones. Exercise floods your body with endorphins: the chemicals that cause 'runner's high'. These little dudes improve your body's reaction to stress and enhance your mood—another bonus.

Gyms have their place in body sculpting and fat loss, but they're not for everyone. Luckily, you can move anywhere, anytime. You may believe that exercise and fat loss can only occur in a gym, but have you heard of the Gym of Life? I've been a member forever. It's free, convenient and it comes to you; no start-up costs, no heckling, no Cardio Queens. You don't need structured exercise if you join. It's all around us and, with a bit of creativity, we can always be active members.

Movement chi

Our bodies convert food to fuel via the energy highway of our body. Every single day everyone creates and consumes an amount of ATP (adenosine tri-phosphate) appropriate to their own body weight. The energy released by that series of reactions is how we convert glucose into energy and what keeps us powered up.

The body has two main energy systems that convert food into ATP: the aerobic (with oxygen) and anaerobic (without oxygen) energy highways. Energy is needed in order for us to carry out living our everyday lives—without it we wouldn't be able to get out of bed. Energy is needed for exercise, as well as for body maintenance and growth.

NinjaMove

THE 10-MINUTE WORKOUT
When you don't feel like exercising, promise yourself just 10 minutes—a walk, or a stint at the gym. Everyone can find 10 minutes. And the best news? You'll almost always exercise for longer. The first 10 minutes is the hardest but you will pump out 20 easy, maybe 30 and you will feel so good! (This strategy will stand you in good stead for anything you're putting off.)

'Focus on fitness with meaning, not just fat loss.'

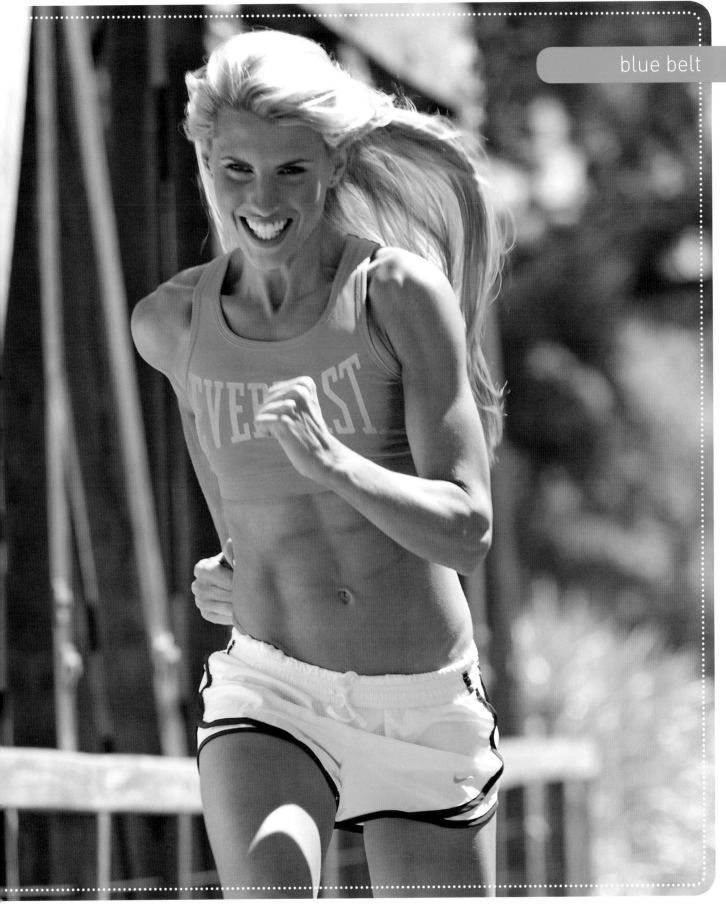

The aerobic energy system is usually the first to be used; when you're active you need more energy to keep you going. When more energy is required the demand for oxygen from the muscles is greater, which makes the heart beat faster and breathing deepen. When the oxygen quota needed by your body can't be filled the anaerobic energy system kicks in. Imagine all these internal processes working away as you walk up a hill or run for the bus. Our bodies are amazingly competent machines and deserve only our respect.

Weightloss warriors know this and focus on the *fit* not the fat: your fitness is more important in gaining the black belt of health and happiness than your weight. If you're healthy and fit you'll look the best you've ever looked in your life. Your goal should be fitness not thinness. (You can be skinny and still very unhealthy with a high body fat percentage, high cholesterol and high blood pressure.) Body confidence comes with fitness, harnessing the power of your hormones and the two main energy systems that drive your body, and not from a thin profile or a small number on the scales. Train for fitness with meaning.

Cardio cheat

There are two types of cardio training: continuous training and interval training. Continuous training is walking, jogging, running, riding a bike or using cardio machines for a specific period of time at an even pace.

Interval training alternates high-intensity exercise intervals with slower-paced periods. Interval cardio helps to burn more calories and fat, improve your cardiovascular fitness, increase your speed and expand your workout options. This method of training is also a great way to increase fitness quickly, zap fat and fit exercise into your busy work day. With interval training being time poor is no excuse. Even 10 minutes will make a difference. Do intervals of walking and running: start by alternating 30 seconds of walking with 30 seconds of running. Do this for 30 minutes. Intervals give the same hormonal benefits and high as excess post-exercise oxygen consumption—after-burn—as longer bouts of continuous intense exercise. We want to be chewing up fat while we train and while we rest.

Add cardio blasts to your circuits. This could be 10 minutes or 30 but make it intense. You could train a circuit in the morning and cardio in the afternoon to maximise the after-burn effect, that way you'll burn calories all day!

The closer you force your heart rate towards your maximum the more your body is forced to use new muscle fibres, which will continue burning calories even during lower-intensity exercise.

NinjaMove

CIRCUITS BY NUMBERS

Try these on for size:
Super 600: 10 exercises of 60 reps each with cardio intervals.
Filthy 50s: 5 exercises, 10 reps each with extended cardio intervals.
Dirty 30s: 30 seconds strength, 30 seconds cardio—alternate cardio intervals.

'Liquid gold' equals intensity

I grew up in a family where sweat was known as 'Liquid Gold'. When we trained together, the first bead of sweat was celebrated with a punch in the air and a shout, 'you're leaking!' Sweating was precious because it meant our bodies were working hard and cleansing.

During exercise your body can burn three possible sources of energy: glucose (blood sugar and sugar stored in the muscles), fat and protein. Protein is the last resort, but whether your body burns its sugar stores or its fat stores depends on one thing: intensity. For intense training, it's easier for the body to use sugar stores as efficient sources of fuel. But this doesn't mean you're burning less fat: by training at a high intensity you burn more calories overall—although your body uses a lower percentage of fat calories to sustain itself through a high-intensity workout it will keep burning more, after, than when you exercise at a more sustainable pace.

When you exercise at a higher heart rate you not only burn more calories during the workout but you boost your metabolism for up to 24 hours afterwards. Now that's worth breaking a sweat for! If you're looking to shed half your body weight or the stubborn 4 kilos you've lost and regained ten times over, the difference is in the intensity of your workouts.

When you sweat, you're training at an intensity that's burning calories and accelerating hormonal benefits. You should be reaching for 85 per cent of your maximum heart rate (220 – age = MHR), in 2 or 3 minute bursts. Intensity will increase your body's release of hormones and train your insides out.

Tiff's Tip

Ban the box. If I turned on the TV every time I got home or woke up, I'd never go for a run. As soon as I get home I put my running gear on and go.

EXERtainment

Try a cardio theatre. There are all sorts of bikes, stair-climbers, treadmills, cross-trainers, walkers, rowers and cross-country machines with screens from bio-feedback to virtual reality, TVs to 'cardio cinemas'. Watching the 6 o'clock news on the treadmill beats the couch.

Get up 10 minutes earlier and move. Walk around the block, do some housework. Just 10 minutes could burn up to 275 calories (1,151 kJ) in a week.

Try a new team sport.

Move to music: Bodypump, aerobics, Taebo, a group boxing class or yoga. Take your friends and make it a date.

Listen to music talking books or a podcast while you walk/run.

Tune in to audio programs or iPhone apps that will coach your training to a new level.

Skipping gets boxers into condition and will get warriors in shape too. Can't beat the convenience— all you need is a flat surface and a rope.

Race a friend on the treadmill, race reps in a circuit, climb stairs in the park.

Add an extra 15 minutes and you could burn up to 100 extra calories (418 kJ) and give your metabolism a stronger boost. Remember, it's all about intensity.

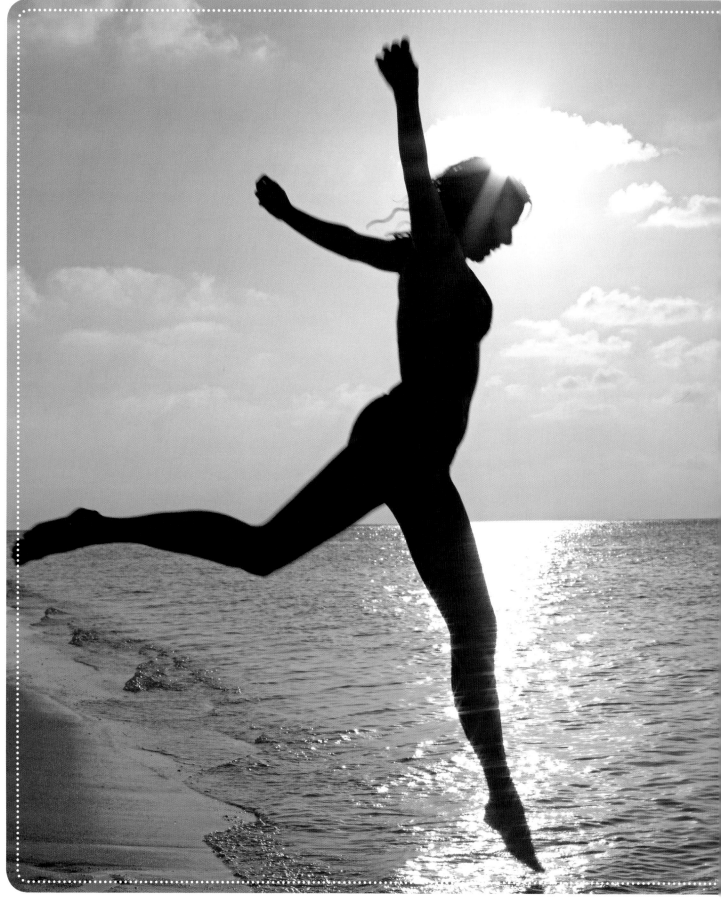

GYM OF LIFE WORKOUT

Walk to the shops. Return your supermarket trolley—I know, this one's a toughie!

Walk quickly, everywhere.

Ditch the car or public transport for the bike, walking—or even running!

Use stairs instead of lifts.

If travelling for business, book a hotel a few kilometres' walk from your office or clients and walk there. Quickly!

Do push-ups in your breaks. Twenty push-ups, five times a day = 500 push-ups a week = 25,000 a year.

Create a walking bus to bring your own and friends' kids home from school.

Don't wait: If you have to stand in line use the time to strengthen your balance and core muscles. Balance on one foot, not two.

MAKEOVER MY WARRIOR WORKOUTS

If you're not getting the results you want, your workout needs a makeover. There are 168 hours in a week. Aim for 5 hours (in 1-hour or ½-hour slots) of sweaty exercise weekly. You'll benefit after only 3 weeks of training.

Muscle in on strength: Chicks who lift moderate-to-heavy weights produce more active growth hormone after their workouts and for a longer time than those who don't. Remember that burger you could burn off while you sleep for every kilo of muscle you build! Find a trainer to teach you correct technique.

Smash the scales: Scales are one way to measure weight loss, but they don't show fat loss. While a kilo of muscle weighs the same as a kilo of fat the volume is different because muscle is denser than fat. That's how two people who weigh the same can look so different. So skinny minnies can be unhealthier than bigger chicks. Always concentrate on fat percentage: for chicks aim for 17-25 per cent, for dudes 17-19 per cent.

Circuit training is the biggest winner: Each circuit station should be a combination of cardio and strength training. Combine squats with sprints and shoulder presses with boxing. Repeat each set three times then move on to two other exercises that work two different parts of the body. Voila! Circuit training.

NinjaMove
GET MOVIN'!
Swap your car for a bike on weekends. Swap self-consciousness for self-belief. If everything jiggles when you're running—embrace it. If it's moving, it's losing. Gotta love that! Swap a dinner date for an active date. Picnic with healthy food, go for a walk—mobile catch-ups or meet friends in a park with the dogs. Swap your couch for a treadmill—watch your favourite show on the run.

Tiff's Tip
ULTIMATE FAT BURNING INTERVAL = 2 minutes on, 1 minute rest.

Metal myth-busting

Myth 1: Weights make a she-man

Okay, so I get that pressing the steel will boost my metabolism and burn muscle, but will I look 'bulky'? When we think 'muscles' Arnold Schwarzenegger's usually come to mind. But working your muscles isn't about becoming brawny, bulky or looking like a body builder. By focusing on the right muscles you'll never add bulk. Instead you'll lose those tuckshop arms, cankles and back cleavage and kick off the growth you need to help burn extra calories. Best of all? You don't need a gym membership or expensive equipment to see the benefits of adding muscle. You can do it with the one piece of gym equipment you already own—your body.

Judging by how often I hear people worry that working out will make them big, they must think that building muscle is easy. Body builders eat and train in a very specific way to look the way they do—none of which we will be doing. Weightloss warriors focus on weight loss and creating a lean healthy physique. Despite my reassurance it's almost universal that ladies worry about looking 'bulky', but because we have less of the muscle-building hormone testosterone it's damn near impossible for us to bulk up. Personally, I'd be more worried about looking bulky through fat than lean muscle.

Here's the thing: after my knee reconstruction in 2005 I've kept up with weight training. Since then I've only built up a slight amount of muscle, even with a personalised training program, specific nutritional plan and professional advice. I'm the same size and weight I was before the op but I have a lower fat percentage, and guess what? I'm still trying to add lean muscle to tone my body more as a lean, mean, fat-fighting machine than a fat-absorbing sponge. While muscles do create body shape, they also give us the metabolic ability to burn calories every time we move; during exercise, gardening, watching TV, even driving. The true advantage of muscles is that they constantly devour calories, even when you're moving 'at the pace of a thousand turtles,' as my grandfather would say. Every kilo of muscle burns between 80–400 more calories (335-1,674 kJ) a day just to sustain itself. Every half-kilo of fat feeds on only 1 to 3 calories (4-12 kJ) to sustain itself. Day after day this is a huge difference in your metabolic rate and daily energy burn. Muscles are the greatest weight-loss investment you can make for the future.

You won't wake up one morning with massive traps and biceps. If anything, a bit of muscle will decrease your measurements. Increasing muscle mass requires diligence. If you do resistance training, using your body as a gym—dips, push-ups, chin ups, jumping lunges and sit ups, and mix up these exercises with a few free weights—your body shape will begin to change. But ladies, I promise there'll be no body builder in sight (unless you start dating one!).

NinjaMove

TRAVELLING

When you're travelling and stuck in a hotel room, ring ahead and ask them to clear out your minibar, then pull out your rope and skip out all your stress. Bring up your knees to increase the intensity. Even if you only have 5 minutes to exercise—run for 5 minutes but make it intense. You may only burn 150 calories (628 kJ) but you'll burn a further 200 calories (837 kJ) from the metabolic boost and after-burn.

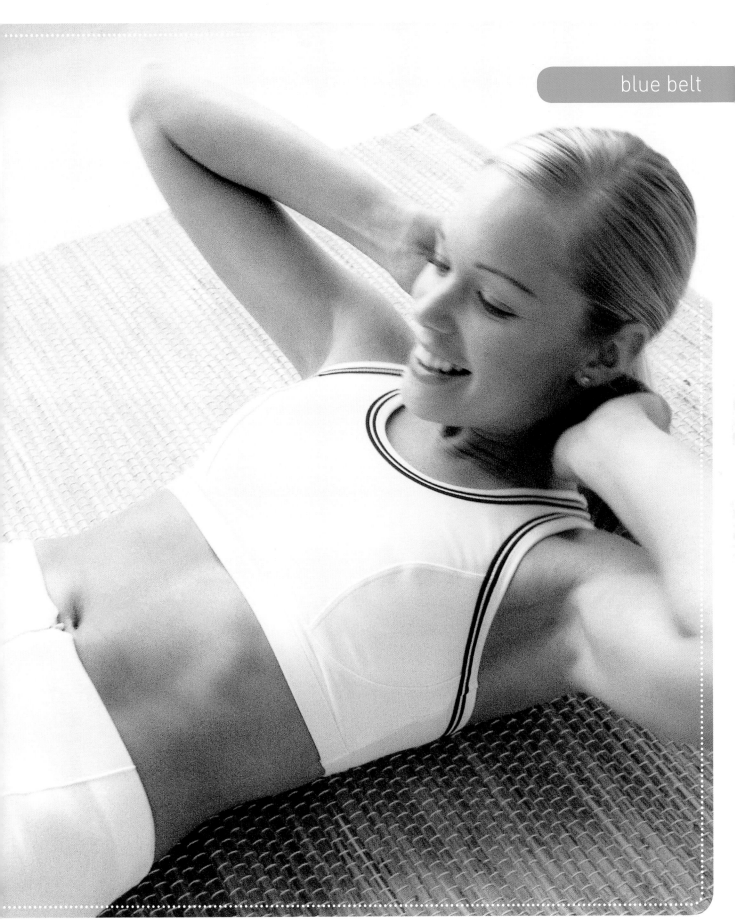

Myth 2: Muscle turns to fat

Weight training helps you build lean muscle to burn fat, but you might worry that if you stop, it'll *turn* to fat. Forget it. Muscle can't change into fat because fat and muscle are two different types of body tissue. If you stop lifting weights your muscles will shrink back to their original size, partially or completely, but they won't turn into fat. If your muscles shrink and your body fat increases from eating too much it might *look* like the muscles have turned to fat. Professional athletes often train and compete for hours every day, burning massive amounts of calories. Michael Phelps chomps through 12,000 calories (50, 232 kJ) a day when he's swimming, but if he retired and kept eating like that he'd have a huge calorie surplus. The result would be dramatic and rapid fat gain—which looks like his muscles have 'turned to fat'.

Myth 3: AB-bracadabra

You can't get a six-pack by waving a wand and chanting 'abracadabra!'
Like many of us I went through the phase of ab crunching every single day, striving for a six-pack. I thought abs were all about training until I realised abs are actually about nutrition. The trick to a six-pack is eating naked. We all have a chiselled six-pack, it just depends on how much warrior padding you wear around your middle. Your stomach is the first place on your body to reflect what you eat, so if you eat naked your stomach will always be flat.

Training your abs every day won't burn more fat, in fact, abdominal training has nothing to do with fat loss. Unfortunately, you can't spot reduce fat. Abdominal training develops the muscle underneath the fat but doesn't remove the layer of fat that may be hiding those washboard abs. You can train your abdominals like any other body part, at most twice a week. They need recovery too. But incessant crunching will not get you a six-pack, nor will any infomercial apparatus, fat burner or product.

If you want a six-pack, commit to eating naked long-term and buying healthy food from your local shops. Eating naked consistently will keep your body fat percentage low and eventually those lines will start appearing. You will also save money by ignoring six-pack exploitation from a diet industry trying to coerce you into buying ineffective products.

Tiff's Tip

The exercise you do today might not work as well in 3 weeks time. You'll need to keep upping the ante.

TEST YOUR FITNESS

Push-up test

Do as many push-ups as you can military style or bent-knee position until you reach failure or exhaustion and count your repetitions.

Results:
30–37 push-ups = excellent
23–29 = above average
12–22 = average
6–11 = below average
5 or less = train harder!

Sit-up test

Lie on your back, knees bent at right angles, feet flat on the ground. Rest your palms on the top of your thighs then squeeze your stomach, push your back down flat and sit up high enough for your hands to slide to the top of your knees.

Results:
33–43 sit-ups = excellent
26–32 = above average
19–25 = average
15–18 = below average
14 or less = train harder!

Squat test

Stand in front of a chair and squat down to touch the chair before standing back up.

Results:
33–43 squats = excellent
26–32 = above average
19–25 = below average
18 or less = train harder!

INTERVAL TREADMILL TRAINING WORKOUT

You can do this interval workout on any cardio machine by alternating the effort levels. Try the stepper, cross-trainer, bike or the rower. Adjust speed and resistance to suit you.

WARM UP: 2 minutes at 3–4 km/h or at a pace where you can talk easily.
Speed up: 1 minute at 5–6 km/h or at a pace where it's hard to talk.

1. Tough
Speed up: 2 minutes at 6–8 km/h or at a pace where it is impossible to talk.
Slow down: 1 minute at 3–4 km/h or to your comfortable walking pace.

2. Tougher
Speed up: 2 minutes at 7–8 km/h or at a pace where it is impossible to talk.
Slow down: 1 minute at 3–4 km/h or to your comfortable walking pace.

3. Even tougher
Speed up: 2 minutes at 7.5–8 km/h or at a pace where it is impossible to talk.
Slow down: 1 minute at 6–7 km/h or at a pace where is hard to talk.

4. Toughest
Speed up: 30 seconds at 6–8 km/h or at a pace where it is impossible to talk.
Slow down: 30 seconds at 5–6 km/h or at a pace where it is hard to talk.

5. Tough
Speed up: 30 seconds at 6–8 km/h or at a pace where it is impossible to talk.
Slow down: 30 seconds at 3–4 km/h or to your comfortable walking pace.

COOL DOWN: 2 minutes walking.

Weapon of mass reduction:
heart-rate monitor

Ladies, the Weapon of Mass fat Reduction fits in your bra! It's the heart-rate monitor. You won't know your fat-burn rate until you wear your heart monitor for 3 days straight. Take note of how many calories it takes to bring the shopping in from the car, to walk up some stairs, to jog for 5 minutes or take a group exercise class at the gym. You may think you're working hard but until you see those heart beats click over those calories, you won't understand how hard you actually have to work to burn off a single 500 calorie (2,000 kJ) muffin. It takes an hour of running flat stick! You'll soon see which exercise elevates your heart rate and works most efficiently for your body. My heart hates hills, kicking drills and first dates—go find what makes yours flutter. In the weightloss warrior's artillery the heart-rate monitor is one of the most lethal weapons.

Don't Zen out or rest between sets of exercises, stay active to keep your heart rate up. The harder the heart beats the more calories you burn. The best kind of active rest is working a different muscle group. If you've been running, do push-ups. Shock your body. Shock = intensity = higher burn.

You can maximise your results by splitting your workout into two separate sessions. For example: resistance train in the morning and cardio train at night—this means you'll burn calories all day. For hours afterwards your body will burn up to 25 per cent more calories by elevating your basal metabolic rate. After-burn is also referred to as 'excess post-exercise oxygen consumption' or EPOC. This is your body trying to restore itself after exercise. By splitting up your cardio and strength training you'll reap the benefits of double strength fat-burn after battle without over training your muscles.

If you don't have time to train twice a day don't fret, once will still get your Active Zen on.

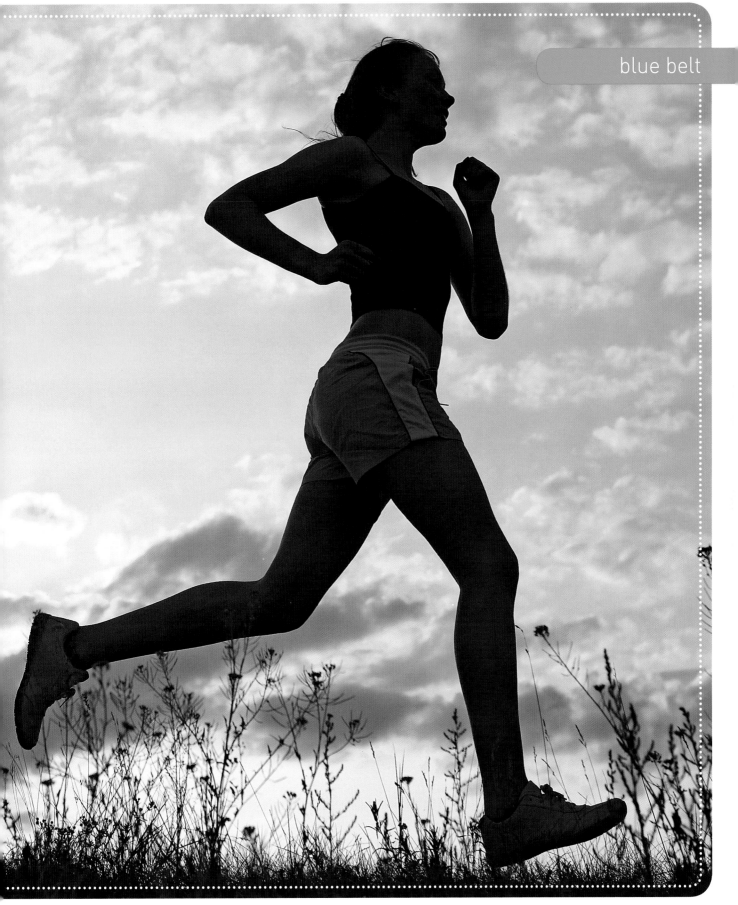

30 ways to burn off a chockie bar!

Scoff an average 50 gram chockie bar and you'll eat around 267 calories (1,117 kJ). But if temptation is just too much you can always hit the gym, dojang, park or yoga studio. Here are 30 ways to burn the chockie off.

Activity	Minutes to burn off chocolate bar (50 gram)		
	60 kg person	80 kg	100 kg
Running up stairs	19	17	15
Running	27	24	21
Step machine, moderate intensity	31	27	24
Cross trainer, moderate intensity	35	31	27
Cycling	35	31	27
Touch football	35	31	27
Martial arts	40	35	31
Football, social game	40	35	31
Paddle surfing	40	35	31
Rowing machine, moderate intensity	40	35	31
Swimming	40	35	31
Basketball, casual	46	41	36
Boxing	46	41	36
Netball	46	41	36
Mowing lawns	50	44	40
Baseball	55	49	44
Dancing	62	54	48
Walking outdoors	63	55	49
Golf game, no buggy	64	57	51
Aqua aerobics	69	61	54
Gardening	69	61	54
Tennis	69	61	54
Housework	79	70	62
Golf, driving range	92	81	72
Surfing	92	81	72
Volleyball	92	81	72
Weight training, moderate	92	81	72
Walking the dog	99	87	77
Pilates	110	97	87

Sweet dreams

Snack right: Avoid carbohydrate-based snacks before bed, particularly grains and sugars. These will raise your blood sugar and inhibit sleep. Later, when blood sugar drops too low (hypoglycaemia), you might wake up and not be able to fall back to sleep. If you're hungry eat a high-protein snack several hours before bed. This can provide the L-tryptophan needed to produce melatonin and serotonin.

Cut back: Another reason to limit the alcohol: that second wine might make you drowsy but the grogginess won't last. Alcohol fuels a neurotransmitter that helps you feel sleepy but as the booze is metabolised your ever-resilient brain works to rebound and cancel out its sedative effects. By the time your liver has processed that vino your brain has overcompensated leaving you awake and restless.

Switch off: No TV right before bed. It's too stimulating for your brain and will take longer to fall asleep after. Even better, get the TV out of the bedroom or even out of the house completely.

Block out artificial light too. Biologically, we haven't yet learned to distinguish man-made from natural light so any brightness sets off our wake cycles. After hours, illumination also disrupts the brain's nocturnal production of the sleep hormone melatonin. The tiny red light on the TV won't keep you from dozing off but the glow from your computer will. Turn everything off before bed. If you need to go to the toilet during the night, don't flick the switch—the light will perk you up again.

Tuck in: Get to bed as early as possible. Our systems, particularly our adrenals, do the majority of their recharging or recovering between 11 pm and 1 am.

Cool down: As we sleep, our thermoregulation system diverts blood from our core to our extremities, a process that lowers body temperature. This automatic cool-down is an evolutionary response designed to preserve energy for waking hours. Sleeping in a chilly room is optimal and will speed the process along so you fall asleep faster. With a pair of socks you can cause the blood vessels in your feet to expand, encouraging blood flow and aiding your body's cooling mechanism.

To max it out, change it up

Exercise puts stress on the body forcing it to adapt and change. You have to outsmart your body by continuously shaking up your routine. Undulate your intervals, sprint for 90 seconds, rest for 30 seconds until you reach 10 minutes. Or run at a different speed every minute. Do incline intervals, or mix up strength training intervals with cardio intervals. Try 10 minutes of exercise on five different cardio machines. Try a different kind of exercise altogether—go surfing, rock climbing, rollerblading.

To change your body you have to change your exercise routine, and often. Cross training is an excellent way to shock your body and develop different areas of fitness. We allow one set of muscles or physiological system to rest while exercising another, maximising the amount of work we can do and the benefits. To develop speed you may do sprint training and technique drills, then weight training at the gym the next day. By varying your routine you maximise recovery.

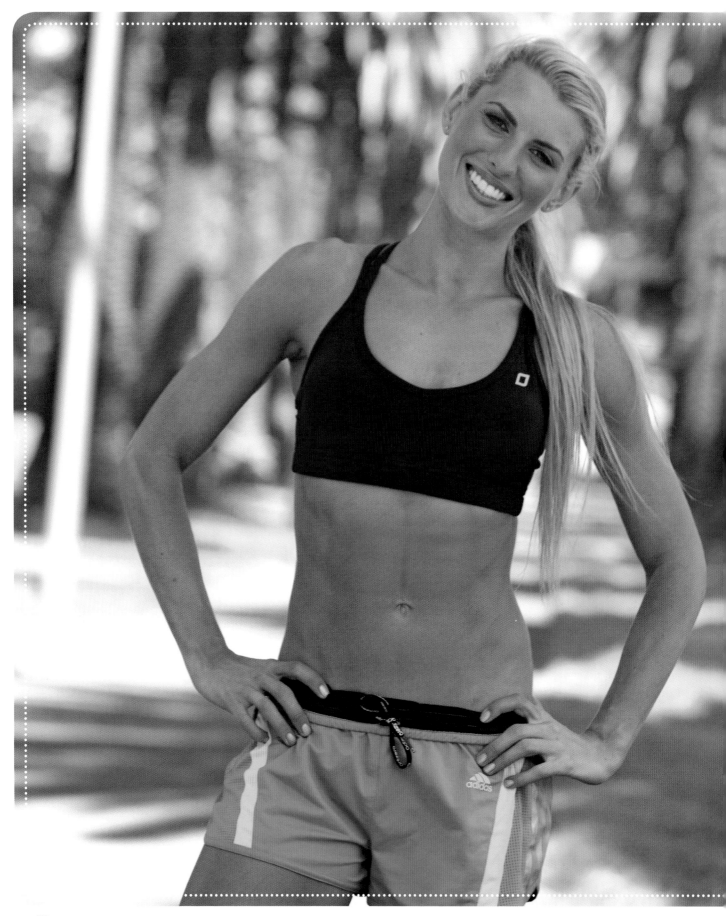

FOREVER FITNESS

Keep a fit log

Keep a fit journal for 4 days a week—2 weekdays and a weekend. Record everything you do and how long it takes. Include housework, travel, even watching TV. It will reveal your priorities, like if you've chosen watching TV over a 30-minute walk after dinner.

Stay strong

Inform others of your fitness goals. Ask them for regular words of encouragement and help: maybe they could look after the kids so you can train. Better still, band together and set fitness goals with your friends. You won't be the only one wanting to be healthier. Instead of catching up for a coffee, catch up for a walk and talk. Go shopping together or get a take-away coffee. Walk with the take-away coffee for 30 minutes in your lunch break.

Add variety

Make exercise a game. List all the activities you love that make you sweat. Include things such as rollerblading, salsa classes, cycling, power walks, hiking, rock climbing, washing the car with the kids. Circus classes, cartwheeling, beach runs—it all counts. Get excited to move. Motion creates emotion. Exercise should come from pride and excitement not guilt. Believe that you deserve to be strong and healthy. If that's your priority it will be easy to get up and GET YA NINJA ON!

iPod your workouts

Have a new playlist for each workout. Choose songs that inspire.

Start the day with movement

Moving first thing—be it a stretch or a run—will boost endorphins, restore your hormones, burn calories and get your blood pumping for the day. You don't have to run kilometres but being active first thing instead of sitting down for a cup of coffee will set you up to be more emotionally fit for the entire day.

Keep on track

If you get a flat tyre you don't stab the other three tyres and give up. Same goes for missing a workout. Everyone needs to recover; everyone has a few bad days. No matter how bad it gets, you can always rediscover the warrior path.

Get a coach

Everyone needs a coach—I have a few! If you make an appointment with someone and become accountable to them for your fitness then you'll show up. Showing up is harder than the workout. Write it in the diary and stick to it. Block out three separate appointments. Even if you don't have a trainer, make the appointment with yourself.

Never binge exercise

If you have a few bad weeks don't plunge into a hardcore exercise program of hours of intense exercise every day. Binge exercise will disrupt your hormonal balance just as much as junk food.

Perseverance

When we are beginning on the road to change we are forming a new relationship with ourselves, we are demanding new things and expecting different outcomes. We flirt with the idea of change for as long as we can. We try to keep the relationship casual for as long as possible while we suss out if we are compatible, until something shocks us into a sense of urgency and we are confronted with commitment. This is the point where many people regress; they regain the weight, find an excuse or retreat to safe old comfortable habits. Don't do it. KEEP YA NINJA ON!

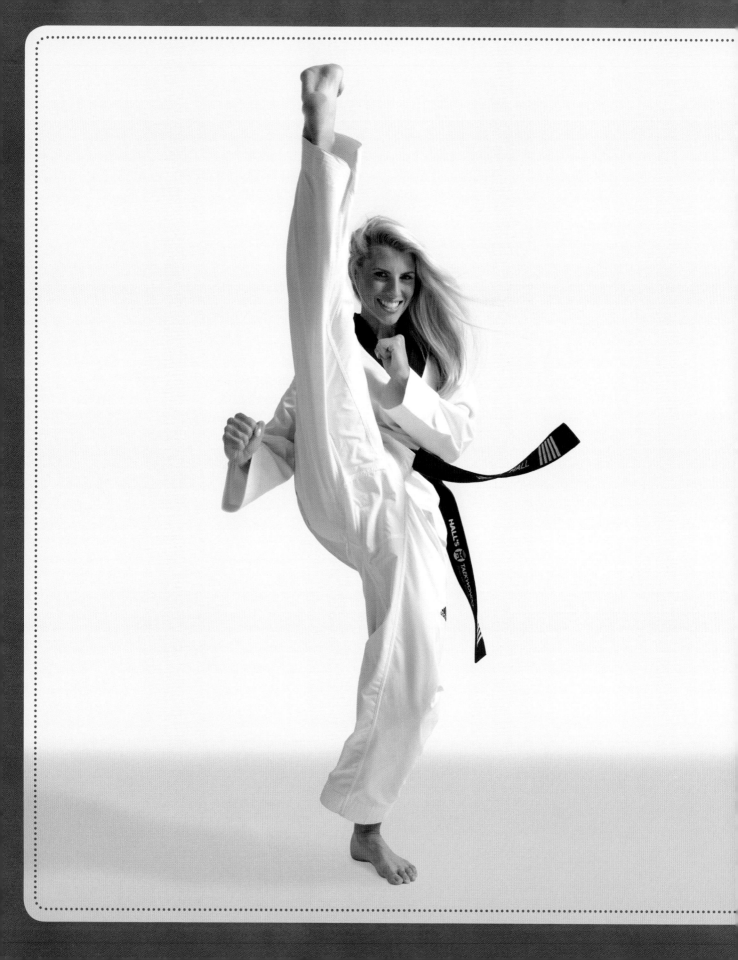

Red belt: Warrior heart

'GREAT WARRIORS NEED THE SUPPORT OF A GREAT TRIBE'

Live like a warrior

NinjaNewsflash

FAT-FREE IS NOT
SO FREE AND EASY

Ninety-five per cent fat-free means
that for every 100 grams of food
you get 5 grams (1 teaspoon)
of fat. Check the serving size: 200
grams of 95 per cent fat-free food
sneaks in 10 grams of fat. Not
to mention the bad sugars that
probably come with it.

Few of us live like hermits, in complete isolation. Most of us have some kind of tribe, whether they're friends, a partner, or extended family. It's important that our tribe supports us in our warrior ways, and if you're a parent you have the additional responsibility of raising the next generation of warriors. When you know how to care for yourself—eating well, moving with pleasure, attending to your emotional needs— you can be an example for your tribe of how to use food for nourishment rather than as a distraction from uncomfortable feelings or boredom.

I've got a message for frantic warrior mums: put yourself first for once. Mums can be the busiest warriors in battle, spending most of their time looking after their tribe and not enough time taking care of themselves. When you have kids, it's hard to find the time to focus on yourself and when you do, you may feel guilty. But your health must come first. Just as in the safety video on board an aircraft—where you have to 'Fit your own oxygen mask first before assisting others'—you have to look after yourself so you have the passion and vitality to then train your little ninjas.

By raising your children as health ninjas you are teaching them skills they'll carry through their whole lives. The ultimate motivation to achieve long-term weight-loss success is family. Because you know what? Health and quality of life is not just about you. You are the Warrior Goddess of your tribe—when you tune in to your inner warrior, your whole tribe will benefit.

Weight loss is about connecting to the self, becoming more self-aware and learning about your body, mind and spirit, and how to nurture them. There's nothing wrong with being a little selfish. The only way to lose weight and not have it return is to enlist yourself for the journey, offload emotional baggage, and put yourself first. After all, the better you are to yourself, the better you can be to those you love.

Be your own force-field

Our brains are wired to make us automatically absorb the emotion of the people around us. Negative energy floats through the air—you know it when you see its effects, whether it comes from an impatient bank teller or your clingy best friend. The energy of others affects us without us even realising. Ask yourself: who makes me feel bad about myself? What drains my energy? Take time to notice the chi around you. Negative chi, toxic friends and poisonous relationships will mess with a weightloss warrior's hard-won harmony.

If you spend time with people who nourish your soul and make you resonate with energy, you will feel vitalised to make positive decisions and choices. Now, I'm not promising you'll find Prince Charming, but I will tell you that dreams can come true. Want to wear a bikini? Squeeze into your wedding dress? Waltz into a dress store and grab a size 12? Don't just dream it, do it. You've gotta eat nude food, find your fire, and rally the support of your tribe. You don't know how long you'll have to stick at it, so steel your ninja soul.

LEAN ON THEM: YOUR TRIBE IS YOUR SUPPORT

Fight flagging motivation with a phone call. When you're struggling, call and talk to a nominated warrior supporter. Tell them how you're feeling, why you're hurting or why you don't know what you feel like eating.

Swap a guilt trip with a pat on the back. Sometimes we need others to remind us how well we are doing and what we have achieved.

Share your discoveries with your friends and family. By helping others we can empower ourselves.

Be honest with each other. If you slip up, don't hide it. Lying about what you eat just makes you feel guilty and sets off a vicious cycle of guilty gluttony or binge eating. Be open about your experiences.

Have a mentor. Everyone knows someone who has achieved something great—be inspired by their journey and one day you may find yourself sharing your journey and inspiring others.

When in doubt, write it down. Writing to your inner warrior (or even to someone else) is a very therapeutic tool. You will learn more about yourself—your habits, your weaknesses and strengths. A journal can serve as a gratitude log to record how far you've come and what you're thankful for.

Find a weightloss warrior pen pal. Get online—it could be someone on the other side of the world who is sharing the same struggles as you. It's sometimes comforting to know that you're not the only warrior worried about your health.

Help, don't hinder, your tribe. Remember to be honest and positive with each other. No one needs 'shoulda, coulda, woulda's in their tribe. Help to lift each other up instead of dragging each other down. Positivity is just as contagious as negativity, but it gets you to where you want to go— one step closer to a black belt in health.

Self-nurture, don't self-torture

The best way to combat cravings and battle binging is to stay in touch with your physical and emotional needs. Healthy self-nurturing is the warrior way to lose weight!

If you are a Diet Devotee, you may have the habit of dieting strictly, breaking the restrictive regime by overeating, then committing yourself to a gruelling diet once again. Deprivation leads to extreme desire to eat whatever it is that you've given up.

Voices make choices

Close your eyes. What do you hear? If it's negative chi thoughts like 'I'm stuck', 'I'm worthless', 'It's too hard!', you're sabotaging your inner warrior. Who is this person who makes you feel you'll never measure up? The answer is YOU. These are the things that you say to yourself. You wouldn't talk to your best mate like this, yet this is how many of us speak to ourselves.

The voice that will combat the haters and silence the critics is yours. Choices create habits, and your inner voice decides which choices you will make. As long as you have a strong inner voice, nothing can break you. But you have to listen and work on making your self-messages positive.

One of my *Biggest Loser* contestants loved to travel. She would fly all around the world if she could, just to escape having to take the most difficult journey of all—the journey of self-discovery. In the dojang she learnt that the greatest journey is the journey into our own heart—no passport, tickets or luggage required! For years she had been running away from herself to avoid having to pause and confront what was making her so unhappy. When we know ourselves, we know how to relate to others. When you change your inner voice, you will change your life.

The most romantic place I've ever visited is in Verona, Italy—the setting of Shakespeare's *Romeo and Juliet*. Juliet's balcony was tucked away in a small courtyard laced with vines and fringed in violet shadows, only accessible through an ancient sandstone archway. Local lore has it that if you write your lover's name on the wall of Juliet's house, you will remain soul mates forever. As you'd expect, the walls and ceiling of this corridor are etched with thousands of inscriptions, the names of lovers from all around the world. I added the name of my boyfriend, confident that he was 'the one' for all eternity. Well, guess what? We broke up as soon as I came back from that trip. Ever since visiting Juliet's balcony, I've wondered about my soul mate, and promised myself I'd return to Verona to scratch out my ex's name and replace it with that of my one true love. Weightloss warriors, I'm here to tell you that I finally know the name I'll write on Juliet's wall, whenever I go back there: Tiffiny. What I know now, that 19-year-old Tiff didn't, is that in a warrior's heart self-love is the foundation for all other kinds of love.

Forget love, I'd rather fall in chocolate

My best friend once gave me a card embroidered with the message 'Forget love, I'd rather fall in chocolate'. I framed the card and hung it up. It's not a slogan you'd expect to find in my house, but I believe it's important to indulge once in a while and for me this usually involves chocolate! But there's a difference between treating and gorging. Sometimes we just need to fall a little in chocolate.

Did you know chocolate was once the food of choice for wisdom-seekers? It's made from cacao beans from the theobroma tree; 'theobroma' means 'food of the gods'. Since chocolate was once revered by the ancient Aztecs and eaten only by those needing wisdom—warriors, noblemen and priests—it's no wonder chocolate feeds the ninja soul. Pure chocolate is bursting with antioxidants called flavonoids, which can help to prevent a whole heap of diseases. And good quality chockie is packed with nutrients like iron, calcium, magnesium and vitamins. But in this nude state, chocolate is very bitter, so most of the bars we buy have sugar and milk added to make it more palatable. Rather than encourage our sweet tooths, if you're going to indulge in a little choc therapy, make it dark and at least 70 per cent cocoa.

NinjaMove

MY CAKE CREDO

More air means fewer calories so if you choose to eat cake, pick one that is spongy rather than dense. Lamingtons are a good choice because they are airy, only lightly dipped in chocolate, and come in small fingers so it's easy to control your portions (20 gram lamington = 45 calories (188 kJ)).

HOW TO BE A CHOCOLATE NINJA

At Easter opt for small, hollow or mini eggs to limit your intake. Or try a bar of chocolate. If you're the type that can stick to a few squares at a time, then you won't go too far off track.

Gradually wean your taste buds on to a darker, good quality brand of chocolate that has a high cocoa content (at least 70 per cent). Only enjoy white or milk chocolate occasionally, as they don't have the same health benefits. Shop at health food stores for healthier, organic chockie.

Drink cocoa made with skim milk to satisfy your chocolate craving.

Indulge in chocolate-dipped fruit like strawberries, blueberries and nuts such as almonds or walnuts. This way you'll get the taste with fewer calories and fat, while also amping up the antioxidants!

Tiff's Tip

Deprivation creates a starving-then-stuffing cycle.

As long as you are treating and not gorging, eating out of pleasure and not pain, then it's okay to eat chocolate mud cake occasionally. Eat it out of love and choice and know that your healthy and fit body will burn it off. That's ecstasy!

Sometimes I need to feed my soul and not my body. Sometimes I want to forget everything I know about hormone harmony and metabolic burn, and just savour how beautifully the silky mint slice melts on my tongue. But the key word here is 'sometimes'. So when you decide it's time, eat without guilt. Eat consciously, slowly and whole-heartedly, while you fall in chocolate.

NinjaMove

AVOID THE ARTIFICIAL
Always opt for foods with the least number of artificial sweeteners, flavours and colours. Artificial colours interfere with your kids' metabolism. The worst are blue 1 and 2, green 3, red 3, and yellow 6. Choose colour-free medication and treat your kids with real ice-cream rather than icy poles.

WHAT MAKES ME HUNGRY?

My empty stomach—hormones in my stomach will alert my brain that I need to eat if I have skipped meals or if I'm fad dieting.

Eating—alerts my brain to the presence of food and makes me want to indulge.

I see and smell food—this makes me want to eat with my eyes when often I am not listening to my stomach that is already full.

I'm stressed and emotional—50 to 80 per cent of eating is non-hungry eating. Knowing that food can calm and numb my pain makes me crave it at times of emotional upset.

Skipping meals—eating small, well-portioned meals every four hours or so will keep my blood sugar levels stable so that they don't drop so low that I feel famished and eat in an out of control way.

Not eating the right food combos—I buy myself an extra hour of satiety by eating a combination of protein, good fat and fibre-rich carbohydrates.

Under-eating—I know that if I don't get enough food I will trigger starvation mode, get hungry and eat the wrong stuff.

Emotional hunger—I take time to find out the triggers and reasons I turn to food when I'm feeling upset or stressed out. I know I must heal these issues. There is no need to take it out on my body.

Physical activity—physical activity will at first increase my appetite, but not so much that the calories I take in will end up being more than the calories I killed in my session. Exercise suppresses and regulates appetite in the long run.

Eating too quickly—it takes 20 minutes for my brain to receive the 'I'm full' signal. In the interim, my appetite may be voracious. I always use the 20-minute rule and apply the brakes on my eating to allow my brain to catch up with my body. After 20 minutes, if I'm still hungry, I'll drink some water (my thirst may be disguised as hunger). If this doesn't work, then I eat a healthy snack.

Shut-eye—a good night's sleep helps to prevent the disruption of hormones that control my appetite. Make sure you wind down before bed with half an hour of 'transition time'—a bath, a stretch, some reading or meditation.

Tiff's Tip

Be your own best friend—
would you speak to someone
else like that? Write yourself a
fan letter. Just try it, no one
needs to read it.

THE 10-MINUTE WARRIOR SPA

Breathe in, breathe out: Take five deep breaths: in through your nose, out through your nose. This relieves stress and gives you a chance to regroup.

List two things you love about your bod: This gives an instant boost of confidence. Positive self-talk is important to keep you on track to make choices that support you, rather than hurt you. The better you talk to yourself, the better choices you will make.

Get fishy: Pop a daily omega-3 supplement to halt winter colds and improve memory and concentration.

Put a cap on it: Swig a cap of flaxseed oil to heal injuries, boost fertility, get your essential fatty acids and decrease inflammation. As well as being good for clear skin and soothing sunburn, it's also brilliant to moisturise your hair.

Go green: Green tea burns up more fat and improves your breath. It's also proven to reduce your weight with healthy eating and exercising—by 5 per cent in 3 months. It also contains a powerful dose of antioxidants so is great for anti-aging. A wet winner!

Gobble a grapefruit: Grapefruit is the new kid on the block for anti-aging. It's vitamin C content boosts collagen production, keeps skin firm and protects it from environmental damage.

An apple a day—Nanna was right! Apples help prevent acne and skin inflammation (your skin is 15 per cent of your weight so look after it!).

Just move: Apply what you learned in high school physics—a body in motion stays in motion. Keep yours moving if you want a long life.

NinjaMove

EAT OUT LOUD

Writing what you eat is the best way to work out what is filling out your jeans. If you're eating 3000 calories (12,558 kJ) a day but only burning 800 (3,348 kJ) of them, eating out loud will show it. An extra 1000 calories (4,186 kJ) a day equals a kilo of weight gain each week. If a food journal isn't your bag, join a food-watching online forum or 'fess up over lunch at work with a designated Calorie Colleague. Understanding your movement chi and food chi is the best way to win the weight-loss battle.

DUCK THOSE CEREAL PESTS

Most cereals are nothing more than confectionary. Even the healthy ones contain a lot of sugar (avoid any cereal that lists sugar in the first three ingredients). And some 'natural' mueslies contain up to 20 per cent fat and 25 per cent sugar.

Learn the label lingo and always look for less than 5 grams of sugars, less than 200 calories (837 kJ) and at least 5 grams of fibre per serve. Low-calorie cereals are often high in sugar, which means you'll be snacking by 10 am. Also aim for low-sodium cereals, where possible, and avoid muesli clusters—sure, they're crunchy and yummy, but also full of added oil and sweeteners.

Good cereal should be based on wholegrain oats or wheat. Untoasted varieties are best, and you can stir in flaxseed or nuts to boost the protein and good fat content. Also, when a cereal claims to contain fruit, make sure it's the real deal, not just reconstituted fruit concentrates and purees.

How to avoid snacking on your feelings

So you've been acing it—drinking water, exercising, eating naked and feeling great. Good on you! Then something happens: a family crisis, a bad day at work, a fight with your partner, or just a mega-dose of PMT. Suddenly you start being more naughty ninja than weightloss warrior. Don't beat yourself up; there will be times when you can't control yourself. Repeat after me, 'No ninja is perfect!'

You're human and humans can be super-emotional creatures, chicks especially. After hoovering everything in the pantry, then wallowing with a massive food hangover, you swear you will never do the Food Frenzy again. But sometimes we'd rather feed on our feelings than allow our emotions to eat away at us. Why? Because hunger is often the last cause of a Food Frenzy. The way to solve it is with one simple question: 'Am I hungry or am I hurting?' To combat the frenzy, the first step is to know your hunger type.

Hungry in the heart

You don't need food, you need a punching bag. You're upset, angry, frustrated, lonely or hurt. You may need a therapist, but you won't find one in the fridge. Combat heart-hunger by tapping into the motivation and support of your warrior tribe and friends. Admit that you are struggling and ask for help. Call a friend or a family member and talk it out. Dump the weight on us, not on your hips.

Hungry in the head

You're bored. You're at a dull work function so you're eating all the finger food. Or you're watching TV and there's nothing on, so you start grazing. Or you're close to deadline, but you just can't motivate yourself. Combat head-hunger by bypassing the danger zones. If there's nothing on TV, turn it off. If it's not mealtime, don't hang around the kitchen. Break the unconscious association between location and eating, whether it's the lounge room, the home or work kitchen.

Another good strategy is to hit the footpath for a walk around the block or even just to check the mailbox. Not only will movement shift your focus but it will also suppress your appetite. Or just get busy. Assign yourself a task—anything from reading a book chapter, to grooming the cat, tackling the Tupperware drawer, dusting the skirting boards or plucking your eyebrows (just don't go tweezer-crazy!).

Hungry in the guts

This is true hunger—your body needs sustenance. You feel empty, dizzy and your belly feels like it's eating itself. First drink some water—often thirst feels like hunger. If you are dehydrated, your cravings will be stronger. You need to eat, especially if you've been skipping meals. So eat. But eat the right food in the right amounts—go for a healthy protein-rich meal or snack. If you're this hungry, stay away from the fruit bowl, as fruit can make you hungrier.

NinjaMove

DON'T PARTY ON YOUR OWN
One of the greatest shocks when I stayed with my *Biggest Loser* family was that they ate party food every day. Family blocks of chocolate, party pies, family packs of Doritos, soft drinks, popcorn—they ate treats like food. If there is a party, then enjoy it with a party treat. But just you in front of the TV, elbow deep in a bag of chips, does not classify as a party. So don't keep junk in the house, don't buy junk, and don't eat junk at home. Party foods are for parties.

'Self-love is like bread,
it has to be made
fresh every day.'

Love bites

Be honest: are you growing a relationship gut? Harbouring some love chub?

Falling in love can make you feel all soft and gooey on the inside, but you don't want to end up with a Lover Layer on the outside. Skip a workout here, order some greasy take-away there, and before you know it, you have more than just butterflies in your stomach—you've got muffin top or beer belly! When we get comfortable in a relationship we make new habits with our new love that can wear away our formerly Sexy Single bods.

You eat out more often

Once you're attached, you want to go out and spend time with your new sweetheart, right? You're sharing everything, so how can you resist sharing ice-cream on a long walk, luscious pancakes at a leisurely breakfast and a giant popcorn at the movies. Couples bond over food, and enjoying it becomes a sensual ritual in the relationship. That's fine—but watch out when eating out. The average restaurant entrée contains 867 calories (3,629 kJ), and that doesn't include mains, sides, desserts or the calories you eat off your darling's fork.

Cupid's fat fix: eat in more often. Cook up the love in the kitchen. Preparing food at home is sensual, especially when you take turns tasting it. Plus, of course, you control the fat and calories. When you do eat out, munch a healthy snack that contains protein and fibre a few hours before your meal. Starving yourself in anticipation of a love feast provokes the starving/stuffing cycle and could lead to after-dinner bloat. Not the best start to a sexy evening!

The horizontal life

Have you been spending too much time in bed or on the couch—anywhere but the gym? Couples who live together for 2 or more years are less likely to be physically active, and the women are more likely to become overweight. As positive as relationships can be, they also change your routine. You schedule more couple's events and have less time for yourself. Drinks with your new squeeze or a date with the old treadmill? It's not exactly a tough choice.

Cupid's fat fix: move together. People who exercise with a partner lose more weight than those who sweat solo. When couples move together, they're more likely to stick with it. Sign up for a fun run, join a gym together, ride a bike, go swimming—do anything that doesn't involve the remote control.

Tiff's Tip

Treats are treats; take the occasional out of it and it's a heart attack waiting to happen.

NinjaMove

TRICK YOUR TASTEBUDS

You can lower your fat content by swapping a few ingredients that don't alter taste but will make a difference to your scales.

Cream—evaporated skim milk;

Milk—low-fat milk;

Sour cream—low-fat yoghurt;

Cheese—cottage or ricotta cheese (awesome in lasagne!);

Mayonnaise—a low-fat variety or low-fat yoghurt;

Salad dressing—lemon juice or vinegar;

Oil/margarine—halve the amount or sauté your vegies in water;

Coconut cream—evaporated low-fat milk and coconut essence.

Bite for bite

Do you have 'portion distortion'? It can be tough for the ladies to stick to petite portions when your dining companion downs 500 –1550 more calories (2,093–6,488 kJ) a day than you do. You no longer recognise a normal-sized serving because you're always eating with a guy who consumes mountains of food. He might be able to get away with it (guys have more muscle mass, so they require more calories), but matching him bite for bite will make you stack it on.

Cupid's fat fix: serve yourself smaller amounts of food. Use a side plate for yourself and a dinner plate for him. Chicks burn 26 per cent fewer calories than blokes, so at that rate you'll just about break even.

You're happily fat

You have a loving partner, so who cares about the extra 5 kilos? But what's good for your heart may be bad for your hips. Happy people in relationships find it harder to lose weight.

Cupid's fat fix: weigh in often. It's great to accept your body and indulge yourself occasionally, but when all your pants are too tight and you're suddenly flinching whenever your lover's hand strays near your jelly belly, it's time to change. Regular tape measurements or weigh-ins will stop things getting out of control.

Still need convincing? Even small amounts of weight loss can lift libido. Chicks who are more active and happier with their bodies have more satisfying sex lives. Take it off, to get it on!

NinjaMove

FAMILY CIRCUITS

Grab your kids, and some basic equipment—a skipping rope, some cones, balls and hoops—and set up stations in your backyard or a park. Do 2 minutes at each station: skip with a rope, zigzag through the cones, wiggle with a hula hoop, bounce a tennis ball using alternating hands, then finish with a set of star jumps.

NinjaNewsflash

SPEAR YOUR BREKKIE

Asparagus spears are great to start the day with because they reduce fluid retention, the stems are stacked from stalk to tip with nutrients and minerals AND they taste great with rye toast, tomatoes and poached eggs.

ESCAPE THE TIM TAM TRAP

Ever think, 'That first Tim Tam was delicious, but where did this empty packet come from?' Willpower doesn't seem to stand a chance when bickies and other treats trigger the reward centre in your brain that makes you want to scoff more. With the first Tim Tam your brain goes 'yeah, baby!' The more you eat, the more your brain makes a link between chocolate bickies and feeling good. After a while, you munch without noticing, just to shut up your brain's craving centre. That's why the Tim Tam packet is suddenly empty.

Try 'Thought Stopping'. The moment you start to crave, acknowledge your craving, and make an instant decision to say 'no'. Once you begin the 'should I? shouldn't I?' you're already gone.

Tiff's Tip

Give yourself some food rules, like never eating standing up with your head in the pantry, or stocking your cupboard with nuts rather than bickies. Most importantly, become aware of your cravings and when you do eat, eat mindfully.

Ritual renos

With minimal effort, a bit of warrior heart and a lot of passion, you can renovate your worn-out rituals and give your unhealthy habits a makeover. Make a list of what you want to change and brainstorm ideas to reinvent new, more nourishing habits.

Unhealthy habit #1: Your car is your dining room

With a schedule tighter than Posh's designer dress, time behind the wheel may be the only chance you get to eat. Problem is, you can inhale an entire day's worth of calories in one drive-through run.

Ritual reno: fill your glove box with snacks that will make you feel full fast. Nuts are great because their healthy fats/protein combination satisfies with just a handful. Fill some snap-lock bags with small serves to eat on the run. Energy bars also make good portable meals for ravenous road warriors. If you must stop for food, head to the nearest supermarket and pick up a salad, some fruit or a can of tuna in spring water.

Unhealthy habit #2: You drink dinner

It's the perfect way to celebrate Friday, but if you refill your glass too many times, you could end up downing a flood of empty calories.

Ritual reno: if you're planning to party, watch what you eat during the day. Make sure you eat something with quality protein to fill you up and pump up the volume of vegies on your plate. A good option is tuna and salad on a wholegrain roll. And keep hydrated! Water will keep your appetite behaving.

Before you go out, eat a fibre-rich snack. This will slow alcohol absorption, and keep you from ordering a mound of nachos before the barman brings your change. The best choices include spirits with soda water (about 60 calories (251 kJ) per serve), white or red wine (around 85 calories (355 kJ) per 120 ml glass), and light beer (around 100 calories (418 kJ) per bottle). Cut calories in half by alternating each alcoholic drink with a glass of water.

Unhealthy habit #3: You pack it in till it hurts

That whole 'just a taste' advice makes you roll your eyes as you dig into your third piece of a workmate's birthday cake. Occasional gluttony has its place, but an all-you-can-eat-all-the-time attitude can cause indigestion, acid reflux and bloating, not to mention making fat ninjas!

Ritual reno: stuff yourself with foods that contain fewer calories per bite. These tend to have a higher water and fibre content, so they fill you up quicker. Gorge on broth-based soups, vegetable salads (carrots, cucumbers, celery, lettuce, tomatoes, green beans), low-fat yoghurt or cottage cheese, apples and pears, wholegrain cereals with low-fat milk, seafood and lean grilled meats (such as chicken or turkey).

NinjaNewsflash

MISSING MUSCLE MASS
We lose 5 per cent of our muscle mass every ten years after the age of 35. So if you don't continue to build muscle you will have to cut your calorie intake by 120 to 420 each day (502–1,758 kJ) to stay at your current weight. That's another reason to move it like you mean it!

Unhealthy habit #4: You eat all day
For you, chewing is like breathing. You probably lose track of what you've eaten, but all that munching can add up.

    Ritual reno: your problem is more about fidgeting than eating. Drink tea or sparkling mineral water as a calorie-free way to keep your hands and mouth occupied between meals. When liquid won't do, choose healthy snacks that require some work— with pistachios, pumpkin seeds and sunflower seeds you'll spend more time cracking shells than eating. Stockpile other goodies that you can eat in individual pieces, like low-fat, air-popped popcorn or dried wasabi peas.

Unhealthy habit #5: You always buy your lunch
You're always in a rush and grab takeaway lunches on the run.

    Ritual reno: buy a reuseable lunchbox and become a weekday warrior with fantastic homemade lunches and snacks. Pack a healthy punch with nude food from the fridge or pantry. Leftover patties, noodles and slices make easy and tasty lunchbox options.

It's okay to say no

If you're a big-hearted warrior (and I know you are), you'll be challenged by heaps of social situations where you don't want to hurt someone's feelings by saying no. I want to tell you it's okay to say no to others because in doing so you begin to say 'yes' to yourself and to the choices that feel right to you and take you closer to your goals. I know you may feel rude turning down a slice of cake at a friend's birthday party or the finger food at an engagement do, but it is totally fine to say no. Or if you can't, just have a taste, and leave the rest. Use the opportunity to practise your eating awareness, maintain your sense of proportion and savour the flavour of every bite. Here are some things you can say instead of 'No, thanks':

    'Thanks for offering, the cake looks delicious!'

    'Dinner was perfect, I couldn't imagine another bite.'

    'I'll have to try some next time.'

Tiff's Tip
Starving yourself will cause you to stuff yourself later. No breakfast = a starving/ stuffing cycle. Eating breakfast is the right start to stop cravings.

NAKED BREKKIE

Morning munchies that are slow to digest will keep you fuller for longer. Protein such as eggs will keep you full for up to 3 hours.

A power brekkie is a combo of complex carbs (such as rye/spelt/wholegrain toasts), lean protein (like eggs) and healthy fats (such as avocado).

Chase your morning flat white with a couple of glasses of ice-cold H_2O. Your body burns a few extra calories heating up the cold water to your core temperature. This may not make a huge difference, but hydrating your body will. The greatest gift you can give your body is a glass of water as soon as you wake up.

Want metabolic magic? Green tea contains a compound that fires up fat burning. You will torch up to 50 calories with two cups a day—that's over 2 kilos a year. Not bad for a few bags. If you are having trouble getting used to the taste, add honey or stevia to sweeten.

CROCKERY CRACKDOWN

Get it in pro-portion

Portion	Looks like	Portion	Looks like
90 grams meat	a child's palm	1 pancake	a CD
150 grams meat	an adult's palm	1 cup cereal	a fist
½ cup pasta or grain	a tennis ball	1 cup vegies	a fist
1 teaspoon butter	the tip of your finger	1 tablespoon dressing	your thumb
1 teaspoon oil	the tip of your finger	30 grams cheese	four dice
1 tablespoon butter	half a ping pong ball	1 medium fruit	a fist

Banish your fat day now

We've all had them—even skinny chicks have those days when nothing in your wardrobe looks right, when you leave the house with an aura of self-loathing floating above your head, instead of a warrior force-field encircling you. Having a fat day has nothing to do with your body, but everything to do with your mind. Instead of attacking the way you think your body looks, ask yourself why you're really upset. Resolve to solve these emotional issues. Instead of staring at the mirror, still your mind with meditation.

Live in the here and now. You can try saying out loud what you're doing as you do it ('I am hanging out the washing'); it helps to focus on the present. Living in the moment nurtures your warrior heart with self-awareness, which in turn tunes you in to the pulse of your body. Being present in the moment will help to keep you centred and calm, and turn a fat day around.

Take a soul retreat. Spend a few moments on a mind vacation; imagining yourself in a peaceful scene floods your body with chill-out chemicals that reduce stress and boost immunity.

Another trick is to focus on your breath. Take a deep breath in, sip the air slowly and sigh it out. Breath is our body's natural ebb and flow, the tides that wash away the useless energy and bring in fresh air, literally.

Touch and be touched; research shows that babies deprived of touch don't thrive, and we weightloss warriors have a great need to be touched too. Get some hands-on love for your warrior heart however you can: hugs, face-to-face catch-ups, massage or cuddles with your kids or partner.

NinjaNewsflash

ZAP THE ZITS

Teenage skin benefits from a protein-rich diet, so try to add one serve of protein at every meal. At breakfast include eggs, for lunch pack sandwiches with skinless chicken or tuna, and at dinner serve lean red meats or fish. Exercise also helps with regulating insulin levels, which in turn lowers other hormones that exacerbate acne.

Tiff's Tip

Use smaller serving bowls. The bigger the bowl, the more you'll stuff it. Look for plates no more than 25 cm in diameter. Your eyes will adjust to the new portion and so will your stomach.

'You are a gift to your body—when you love your body, it will love you back.'

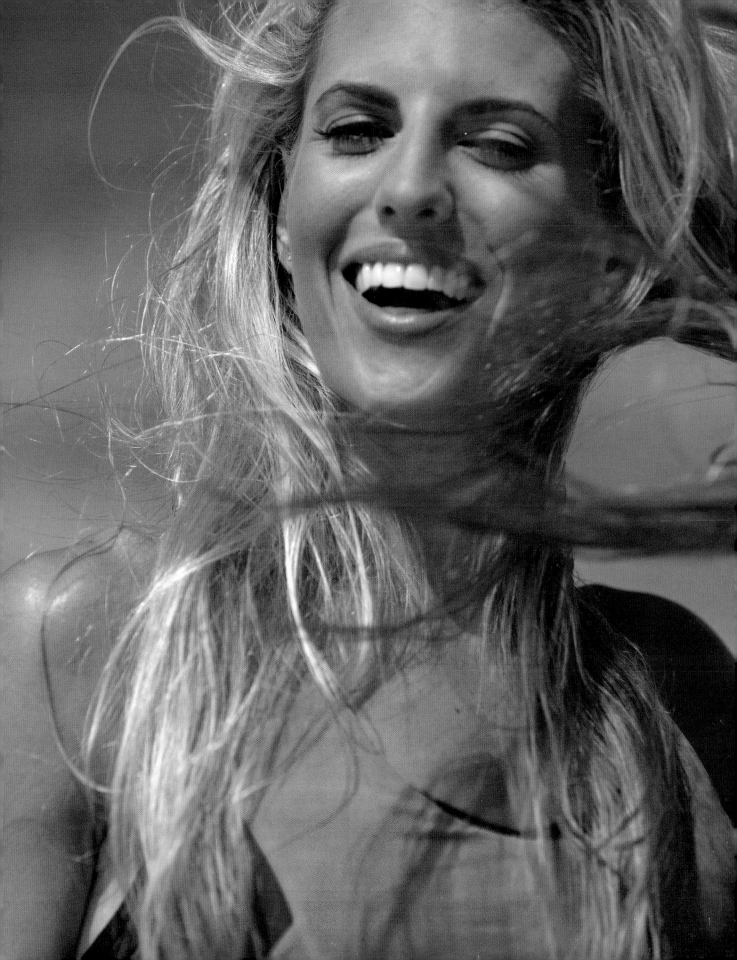

Why additives don't add up

Humans have always needed to prolong the life of food, and this is still true for today's busy, modern households. Traditionally salt, sugar and vinegar were used to preserve meats, fish and fruit and vegetables. These days, food manufacturers rely on more complicated chemicals to keep products fresh and looking glossy:

Preservatives—stop food from rotting quickly

Emulsifiers—keep food textured and smooth

Stabilisers—enhance product consistency

Acidulants—give products a bit of zing power.

Let's look at preservatives first. Preservatives might keep food from spoiling on the shelf but they can spoil your metabolism by disrupting your hormones. Hundreds of foods have preservatives: cereals, baked goods, lollies, alcohol, vegetable oils, chips, some nuts, glacé and dried fruits, chewing gum, processed meats to name a few.

Processed meats especially are packed with preservative. The sodium nitrate in bacon, ham and other deli meat makes it gorgeous pink and prevents bacteria growing. But a diet of hotdogs, bacon and egg rolls and salami pizzas will infect you with the 'slow-metabolism' bug.

The vast majority of food additives are safe, but some are known to cause allergies and other sensitivities and reactions such as asthma, hyperactivity, digestive disturbances or migraines. Australia has had a system of labelling and identifying food additives since 1987. Each additive must be named, numbered and visible on product labels. Eating naked is always safest, but it doesn't hurt to shop smart for the rest of your weekly groceries.

Not all additives are created equal. There are naturally derived additives that we know are okay to eat, such as:

Alpha-tocopherol (vitamin E), which is added to oils to stop them turning rancid

Ascorbic acid (vitamin C), which is used to boost the vitamin content of cereals and fruit drinks

Lecithin (an emulsifier derived from soybean oil and eggs), which is used in baked goods, chocolate and ice-cream.

All of these naturally derived products are classified as 'food additives', even though they weren't concocted in a lab.

Salt—a pinch not a punch

Our bodies only need about 1 gram of salt a day, and the government recommends less than 6 grams of salt a day. The deadliest food a health ninja can eat in terms of salt content is the fast food burger. Last year we chomped our way through 284 million beef burgers—that's 12 burgers each for every man, woman and child. They are so popular it's the biggest rise in consumption across any food group. And we wonder why we're the fattest nation on the planet!

Tiff's Tip

Go for smaller portions of organic and full-fat treats over chemical-laden 'fat-free' ones.

EVIL ADDITIVES

Acesulfame Potassium is a sweetener in gum, soda and baked goods. It has been linked to cancer.

Aspartame (Nutrasweet) is an artificial sweetener in soft drinks, frozen desserts and sugar substitute that has been linked to dizziness, hallucinations, headaches and even cancer.

Butylated Hydroxyanisole (BHA) is an antioxidant in gum, oil and cereal.

Cochineal is an artificial red colouring made from dried insects. Eew! Cochineal can be found in beverages, lollies, ice-cream and yoghurt. Some people are allergic to it.

Fructose is a major invisible fat. Large amounts raise the risk of heart disease.

Maltol and Mannitol are artificial sweeteners used in sugar-free lollies and jams. They have fewer calories than sugar, but are not absorbed well by the body. Large amounts act as a laxative.

MSG (Monosodium Glutamate) is a flavour enhancer used in chips, frozen foods and some restaurant foods. Those sensitive to MSG can experience nausea, weakness and headaches.

Olestra (Olean) is a fat substitute found in some brands of light potato chips that can cause diarrhoea, cramping and flatulence.

Partially hydrogenated vegetable oil is a fat used in biscuits, pastries and ready-made cakes, fried foods, pie crust, shortening and margarine. This is trans fat, a fat foe that messes up cholesterol and your heart health.

Sorbitol is a sweetener and thickening agent that retains the moisture in lollies and chewing gum. Excess amounts of sorbitol can have a laxative effect.

Other additives to avoid: Benzoic acid, potassium bromate, saccharin, sucralose, sodium bezoate, sodium nitrate, sulfites.

Additives to limit: Carrageenan, ethyl vanillin, gelatin, lecithin, mono- and di-glycerides, oat fibre, phosphoric acid, phosphates, potassium sorbate, sorbic acid, vanillin, wheat fibre.

Advancing decoding: For more info on decoding the ingredients list on your favourite products see http://www.foodstandards.gov.au/consumerinformation/additives.cfm

The Hungry Jack's Angus Burger contains 9 grams of salt in the meat patty alone, not even counting the salt in the cheese and the bun! One Hungry Jack's Angus Burger, Hungry Jack's Whopper or McDonald's Angus Burger will exceed your daily salt intake. Why not consider buying low-fat lean mince (about 5 per cent fat) and make your own patties with a wholemeal bun and lots of salad? Better still try my open chickpea burger recipe—it's delicious!

If you're going to use the white stuff—go sea salt instead of table salt, and limit pickled foods, canned fish, tofu, miso, vegetables, sauces and hot dogs. Most of the salt we consume lurks in our breads, so always check the label on your daily bread and go for a low-sodium loaf. To reduce sodium and head off water retention, embrace garlic, lemon, olive oil and pepper. Add herbs and spices to food for flavour instead of salt. Beat-the-bloat spices are cayenne, cinnamon, chilli powder, oregano, ginger, dill, paprika, sage and thyme.

It's time the government introduced 'salt targets'. More than 70 per cent of processed meats, cheeses and sauces contain heaps of salt (sodium). The US and UK have mandatory maximum salt content for their food—let's do it too!

Be a health ninja at the supermarket

A few simple strategies will help you fat-proof your supermarket visits. For a start, always read ingredient labels. Check out the sugar content and select products with lower total sugar. Buy fresh fruit where possible. Avoid fruit packed in syrup.

Cut down on highly processed foods, which are full of sugar. Ignore the pretty packaging and just wheel your trolley past things like prepared baked goods, lollies, packaged desserts, soft drinks and fruit juice. Buy mineral water in preference to sweetened drinks. In fact, see if you can shop around the perimeter of the supermarket, where most of the fresh food is, and avoid the centre aisles, where the packaged and processed foods lurk.

Never shop when you're hungry! Eat before you go, make a list and stick to the items on it. This will help curb impulse buys. Shop at quieter times if you can. Waiting in queues makes you more likely to impulse buy from those tempting checkout displays.

And for the ULIMATE supermarket trick—buy groceries online! If you're not cruising the aisles, you're immune to those enticing in-store displays.

NinjaMove

BREAKFAST AT TIFFINY'S

Eat breakfast every single day. You've been asleep for at least eight hours and unless you can eat in your sleep, you and your metabolism have been fasting that whole time. When you break the fast with a morning meal, you start the fat burning process. But not until you eat. If you don't eat, your body gets paranoid and goes into starvation mode. Your metabolism will start crawling to conserve energy and those extra few kilos will get harder and harder to lose. Not a great way to start a day!

DECIPHERING ENEMY CODES: FOOD LABELS

Fibre—aim for at least 25 grams of fibre per day.

Protein—anything more than 9 grams of protein per serve is considered a high-protein food.

Sodium—aim for 2300 mg of sodium per day, which is equivalent to approximately 6 grams of common table salt.

Sugar—the total grams of carbs in a food serving should be more than double the number of grams of sugar.

Total carbohydrate—this is the sum of complex carbohydrate, fibre and sugars. If the total carbohydrate number is more than double the amount of sugars, that means there are more 'good carbs' than 'bad carbs' in the food.

Total fat—this is the sum of saturated, polyunsaturated and mono-saturated fat (less than one-third of your daily fat intake should come from saturated fat).

Low calorie—anything less than 40 calories (167 kJ) per serve is considered a low-calorie food.

Reduced calorie—this means the product contains at least 25 per cent fewer calories than the regular version.

Light—this means a product has 50 per cent less fat than its regular counterpart. It's better than nothing, but it's still worth double-checking the grams of fat per serve to see what the other 50 per cent adds up to.

Reduced fat—this means that a product has 25 per cent less fat than the regular counterpart (but that could still be quite a lot of fat).

Low fat—this means there are 3 grams of fat or less per serve. Products with this label are usually a good bet.

Fat free—this means half a gram or less of fat per serve, but check for invisible fat (that is, sugar).

Junk-ee rehab

Junk food is like a drug; it's addictive. It doesn't satisfy cravings, it creates them. That's why manufacturers load their foods with sugar, salt and artificial flavourings, and why you should never forget the golden rule: if your food can rot, it's good for you. If it can't go bad, it's bad for you.

Our bodies don't recognise fake foods. Processed foods do not come from nature—they come from factories. Foods high in sugar and unhealthy fats make the brain release endogenous opioids—a kind of biological morphine. Those cream biscuits we're addicted to—with almost 60 per cent sugar and fat—are powerful drug buttons. Just like a drug addict, when you see foods you crave, the orbitofrontal cortex—the centre of craving in the brain—is stimulated. So yes, we can get high on dessert!

When you see junky snack food in packages, you need to look at it not as food but as packaged chemicals. Low-quality starch + sugar + fat + salt + addictive chemicals will never fill you up or help you to lose weight. If you're not eating naked, you're murdering your metabolism. You'll be forever hormonally hungry. Processed food is convenient in the short term, but carrying around excess fat on your body is a massive inconvenience.

Craving combat

Cravings and hunger are different. Hunger is physiological; cravings are psychological, triggered by boredom or depression, or when you see food advertised on TV. There will always be food traps around you and if you're not trained in craving combat it could trigger a binge or a blowout.

When you crave, it switches on parts of your brain that also cause addictions. So reaching for a bong and yearning for Ben & Jerry's 'Berry Berry Extraordinary' activate the same parts of your brain.

You're going to eat treats. It's inevitable. But once you've mastered craving combat you will be proud that reaching for that slice of pizza, is not because you're feeling stressed, lacking control or being a slave to your body's chemistry. You're eating it because it's your choice; you're eating for your body, not from your heart.

Salt: If nothing but the saltiest chip will do, you may have a mineral deficiency. Studies have shown that women who eat low-calcium diets crave salty foods more than those who get enough of this essential bone constructor. One possible reason is that sodium temporarily increases calcium levels in the blood, which tricks the body into thinking the problem is solved. But you may have a shortage of other minerals too.

To combat salt cravings, wet your tongue with a dob of vegemite for a burst of B1, B2 vitamins and salt, or eat a couple of olives.

Chockie: If your idea of a perfect date is an intimate night in with Cadbury in front of a DVD, then you're not just reaching for the chocolate because the flavour makes you swoon, but also because it stimulates the release of serotonin. Chocolate is an antidepressant dessert that your body instinctively seeks out when your happy chemicals are flatlining and need a cocoa defibrillator to jolt them back to life.

To combat chocolate cravings, swap a block of chocolate for a low-fat, low-sugar chocolate mousse. Or whip up your favourite hot chocolate with skim milk or even low-fat custard. Or find a chocolate-flavoured snack bar with high protein and low sugar.

Sugar: Sugar cravings are a lot like chocolate cravings. Lusting after sweets could indicate that you're looking to boost your mood or that you're just low on energy. The body absorbs refined sugars faster than any other type of food, giving you immediate fuel.

To combat sugar cravings, try fresh fruit or low-sugar jelly. Frozen blueberries or raspberries have an additional crunch factor, and fresh fruit with honey and low-fat yoghurt is a satisfying treat.

Sweet and salty: Your body needs glucose and sodium to function properly, so when you get tired you reach for salty–sweet chocolate-covered pretzels to get your cells revving. Combat sweet and salty cravings with peanut butter spread on apple slices, or try a tahini dollop on berries.

Eating through the ages

Surprise surprise! The hot dogs, burgers and deep-fried food you scoffed at 18 don't give you an 18-year-old's body anymore. It's time to learn how to eat right, whatever your warrior age.

20s: Build good habits and bone density by opting for nutrient-rich whole foods instead of refined stuff. Go the apple instead of apple juice and choose wholegrains instead of flour.

30s: Rather than cut out certain foods or reduce calories, eat smaller, more frequent meals that include a balanced mix of carbohydrates, good fats and protein.

40s: To minimise hormone changes that may cause weight gain, replace animal protein and fat with vegetarian sources like nuts, seeds, beans, avocado and quinoa.

50s: To fight stomach fat, focus on swaps. Swap coffee and diet soft drinks for green tea and water. Ditch high-sugar sweets and have dark chocolate or fruit instead.

60s: As your body loses lean muscle, your metabolism slows down and excess weight can creep on. Choose high-quality proteins to maintain muscle mass and your body's natural calorie-burning ability.

RENOVATION TIPS

Spend quality time
Walk on the beach

Go to the movies on your own

Smell your old perfumes—it'll take
   you back to happy days

Build a scrapbook

Take a friend or your partner to the zoo
for a picnic

Potter in the garden

Read a good book

Phone a friend

Linger over a good coffee

Treat yourself
Buy a bouquet of flowers

Invest in new make-up

Indulge in a facial, massage
   or manicure

Try a totally new haircut or colour

Luxuriate with new towels and some
bath salts

Expand your horizons
Enrol in a cooking class

Sign up for yoga class

Take a ride in a hot-air balloon

Try learning a new language

Get away for a weekend mini-break

Honey, I've stuffed the kids

One of the reasons many people say they struggle with their weight is because they were made to finish their dinner when they were kids and that meant eating everything on their plates, even when they were full. I know my friends at school would hide their vegies under their seats and placemats, feed them to the dog, do whatever it took to get out of finishing their dinner. They would be made to sit at the dinner table for hours until every last mouthful of food had been eaten. What they couldn't finish would be packed away for school lunch the next day. When you force kids to eat it interferes with their appetite centres and encourages them to eat when they're not hungry. Don't punish kids for not finishing meals, we're not in a war and that leftover food ain't feeding Africa!

TRIBAL TIPS

Little ninjas (toddlers)

Let the little ones drink only out of a cup or a water bottle—no boxes, cans, cartons or bottles, which all contain added sugar.

Feed kids the same food as adults in the family—it helps to mature their tastebuds.

Don't give up on fussy eaters; keep offering a variety of nutritious foods.

Limit the use of food as a reward or bribe.

Mini warriors (primary school)

Get your mini warriors involved in preparing, cooking and experimenting with food for family meals and school lunches.

Let them shop with you so they see you buying nude food.

Always offer breakfast.

Help them to understand food as fuel and energy; it's not only about taste.

Limit school canteen lunches to once a week.

Growing gladiators (high school)

Gladiators get most of their information from peers and the internet, so it's helpful to talk to them about food and demonstrate healthy eating principles by keeping the pantry stocked with nude food.

Growing gladiators are prone to snack attacks and may eat most meals out. Trust them to (mostly!) make good choices, and make sure you eat naked at home.

Make sure your gladiators grow with protein.

Banish energy drinks from your home and don't buy them when you're out.

Educate your gladiators (girls especially!) about air-brushed beauty. Compliment them on inner, as well as outer, beauty.

Encourage activities like rock climbing, hiking, sport, however you can; offer equipment, transport or moral support from the sidelines.

Be open and honest about the dangers of drugs, alcohol and smoking.

NINJA MOVES FOR EVERY AGE

Little ninjas and mini warriors

Kids this age love to move and it's great for their development.
Try these games in a local park or in your backyard:

- Chasey, running, walking, skipping, sliding, galloping
- Ball games, catching, throwing, kicking, bouncing, hitting
- Climbing, monkey bars, climbing frames, trees
- Digging in a sandpit or the mud
- Racing on bikes, scooters or on foot

- Hopscotch
- Hula hoop
- Frisbee
- Flying kites
- Hide and seek

- Treasure hunts (for girls, raid your costume jewellery drawer for sparkly necklaces as treasure! For boys, mini-dinosaurs or cars)

Teens and twentysomethings

Strength training is very important from the age of 25 onwards. If you want to exercise with your teens or twentysomethings, combine cardio with resistance training. Mix walking or jogging with circuit training by stopping at park benches along the way to do sets of push-ups, dips, sit-ups and squats. Mother–daughter walks are important because 30 minutes brisk exercise a day decreases the risk of breast cancer by 30 per cent.

You could also meet twice a week to train together with a personal trainer (and split the bill!), create a running group with friends, join a local boot camp or sports team together, or take dance lessons together. Setting shared weight-loss and fitness goals—like completing a 5-kilometre swim or a half-marathon—can also get you moving with your tribe.

Golden warriors (Nanna and Pa)

As we age, it's important to maintain muscle mass and flexibility, as these things start to wane over time. For strength exercises opt for elastic bands (like TheraBands) as resistance, rather than traditional weights. Stretching exercises like yoga and pilates are great for building balance and keeping joints moving. The best endurance exercise for golden warriors is water-based movement, which helps to reduce impact on the joints. Go to the pool and tread water, walk laps, do an aqua aerobics class or just swim your favourite stroke.

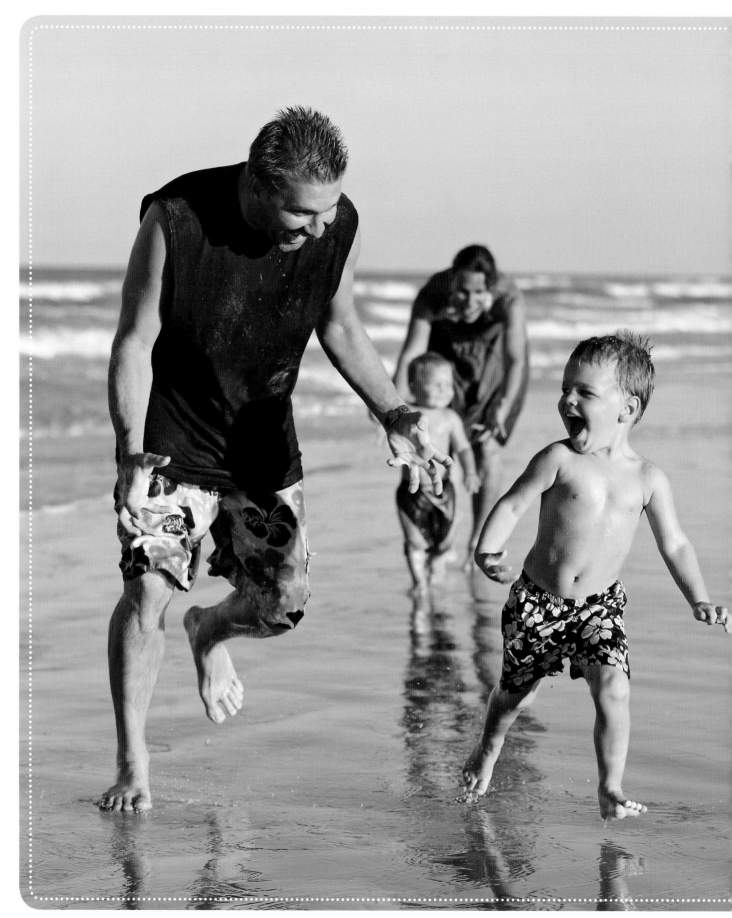

Training your tribe

Time-poor mums have to be stealthy about their weight loss, and even more so when trying to get sullen teenagers or grumpy husbands up and active. The best thing about exercise is that it doesn't have to involve a cardio machine or set of barbells. It can be disguised as play or spending fun time together. The benefits of working out in the Gym of Life include improved self-esteem and confidence. It builds strength and stamina (the fitter they are, the less you have to carry them around). It also regulates your little ninjas' sleeping patterns and appetites, making mealtime and bedtime easier. And best of all, you get in some family bonding time!

THE ACTIVE WEEK

The school run

Create a walking bus and walk your kids to school with their friends.

Drop your kids off early so you can play a game with them in the playground before school starts. A game of football, netball, tunnel ball or cricket before class will increase their concentration for the day.

Make exercise before school a habit: swimming, walks, light jogging or active playtime.

Weekends

Go for a picnic at a local lake, beach or park.

Go indoor rock climbing.

Get involved in a family sport such as martial arts, dance, tennis or football.

Bike ride to brunch at your kids' favourite cafe.

Walk the dog.

Holidays

Ensure family holidays centre around activity and sport: kayaking, water-skiing, surfing, hiking, volleyball, canoeing, camping.

Have fun with beach games: running in the sand, treading water, swimming, body boarding, surfing.

At home

Arm wrestle.

Box with bedroom pillows.

Build a cubby house.

Do active household chores together; washing the car or gardening. Don't make it about the chore but about movement.

Shopping

No matter what age you are, walking several times around a shopping centre is a great way to burn calories and your kids will enjoy it too. Just be clear beforehand there's no stop-offs at fast food outlets as part of the trip!

Walk to the milk bar—the kids can bike, rip stick, scooter, roller blade or skip.

Tiff's Tip

Cutting out processed foods and eating naked is the best way to reduce insulin levels and help control the hormonal imbalances that make zits flare up.

SPROUT WINNING HABITS:
Stealthy vegies for your little ninjas

Stir cauliflower, baby spinach or rocket through your favourite risotto.

Serve carrots with a drip of honey.

Make your own pizza faces using wholemeal pita bread—try lentil, avocado and mixed bean for a vegie delight.

Get stealthy! Blend carrots and stir into pasta sauces, or hide baby spinach in toasted cheese sandwiches and under poached eggs.

If you are desperate—French fry them! Trick your little ninjas by baking fries with sweet potatoes, carrots or parsnips in light olive oil.

Just about any vegie can hide in a Bolognese or lasagne—eggplant, carrots, spinach.

Give yourself a wok-out. Throw together some green vegies and sprinkle with flaked nuts and balsamic vinegar.

SOUPer meals. Light eating makes lighter weight. Try three soup meals a week.

NinjaNewsflash

ACNE ACTIVATORS
Sugary breakfasts, white bread, white rice, chips, potatoes, soft drink, energy drinks

ACNE ASSASSINS
High-fibre, low-sugar, low-salt cereals, rolled oats, sourdough bread, basmati rice, fruit, protein-rich foods, vegetables, unsalted nuts and seeds, sweet potato, water

WIPE OUT WEEKEND WEIGHT GAIN

Stick to a food schedule: Sleeping in, skipping meals, hangovers and socialising can lead to a slump in metabolism. Make sure you get your three meals plus healthy snacks throughout the day.

Plan ahead: Don't start the weekend with bare cupboards; that makes it too easy to eat out or grab a packaged meal. Pay a morning visit to a market, farm store or favourite deli and stock up on fresh ingredients.

Join the Gym of Life!: You don't have to be in the gym to get the blood flowing. Schedule a leisurely walk with a friend, play in the park with the kids, hire bikes or go for a swim.

Choose your fancy: When eating out choose dessert OR wine rather than having both.

Eat in: Bring back the dinner party—it's always healthier than eating out because you can control what you eat and how it's cooked. Plus you get to catch up with your mates!

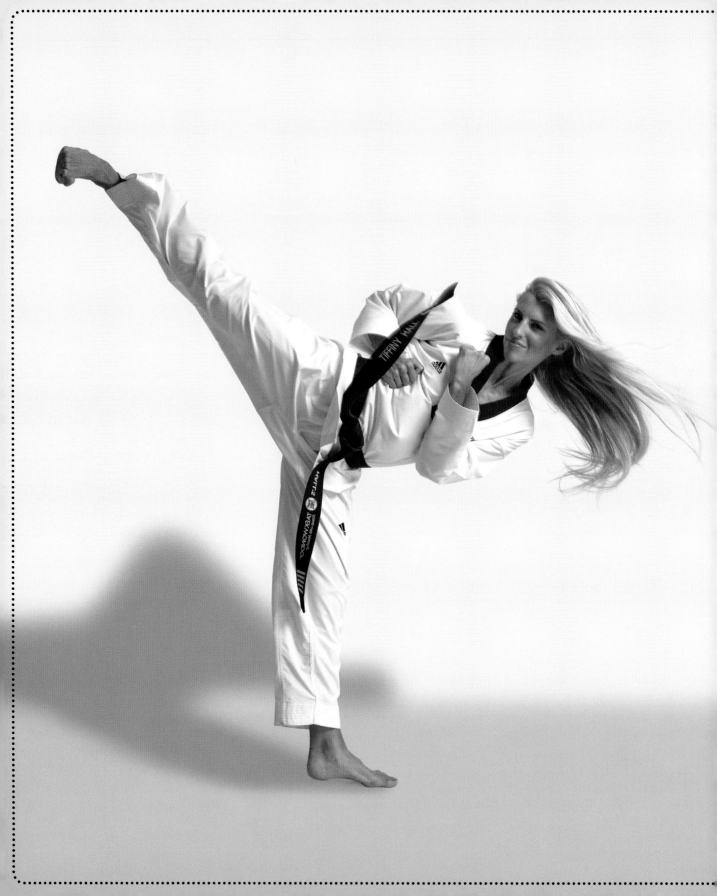

Black belt: Warrior strength

'REAL WARRIORS CONSTANTLY STRIVE TO GROW
PHYSICALLY, MENTALLY AND SPIRITUALLY'

Every ending is a new beginning

NinjaMove

MEDITATE ON THE GO

Exercise can be like moving meditation. Just as yogalates can cleanse your mind, treadmill-ates can also clear away a hectic day. Find your rhythm in your run and take your mind to another place. Pushing yourself in cardio fitness, as with any challenge, requires you to focus and Zen out. If you push to the point of pain and tightness in the chest, you won't last long. Take it breath by breath, just as in meditation, and you will feel yourself releasing.

Welcome to black-belt mastery, my fellow weightloss warriors! It's been a long journey, and it's not over yet. We've travelled many paths, from our minds and bodies outwards to our friends, family and the world. You've come this far, progressed through the white, yellow, blue and red belts and now you stand on the threshold. A black belt in health symbolises self-mastery: the warrior mindset, knowledge about food, hormone harmony and movement chi, and the mental steel to overcome the many obstacles that will appear in your way.

But you're not quite there yet. I've trained plenty of taekwondo students to black-belt level and year after year the hardest challenge I face is motivating them to continue beyond the black belt. Your black belt in health should be both an achievement and an enticement to constant and never-ending improvement. Weightloss warriors must commit to training for life, recognising that obstacles will always exist, and knowing that you have to be nimble, because you never know when the ground is going to shift beneath your feet.

GRAB SOME PRECIOUS YOU-TIME

At work: Give your visitor 2 minutes, then if you still don't know what they want—ask! 'Now, what can I do for you?' steers the conversation straight to the point.

Ditch the lollies from your desk drawer. Ditto the guest chair. Either lose it, or pile it with papers when you really need to work and leave it open when you have time to spare.

With friends: Everyone knows a classic time-sucker—you give them a minute and they'll suck away an hour. Make yourself scarce—decide to make them wait on a reply to their constant SMS, email or phone assault. The time-sucker will still be there tomorrow, even if you don't call them back today.

Do the mobile catch-up: the phone can be the greatest time waster. Use the phone hands-free while you fold washing, cook dinner, walk around the block or do some squats!

At the gym: Knock one or two workouts out of your week. But make the three or four times you do go, longer, harder and stronger. Remember you reap the benefits of your training from both the workout and the recovery.

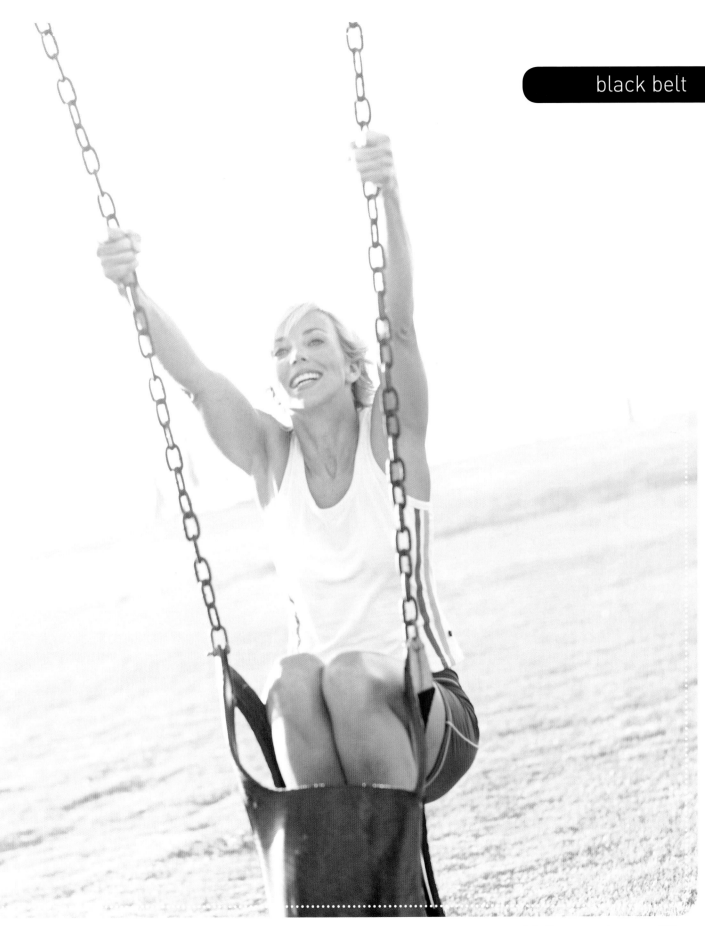

Tiff's Tip

When exercise is nothing but another chore, when work is hectic and there seems no time for health—or looking after yourself—reconnect with your innermost passion.

The meditating warrior

When I suggested to my stressed-out *Biggest Loser* ninjas that they try meditating, they said, 'What's that got to do with burning fat?' They thought meditation was only for Buddhist monks or dope-growing hippies. Think again. Meditation can reduce stress, promote healing, increase immunity and even make you smarter. It also breaks negative thought patterns. Obsessing on the same thought over and over cuts a track in your mind, making it easier to think the same way in the future. In other words, if you always think self-critical and self-defeating thoughts, your neurons get used to firing along those pathways, and those thoughts become a habit that gets harder and harder to break. Meditation provides a technique for retraining our reactions to stressful situations.

Once you meditate regularly, you strengthen your resolve to stop *before* you devour a whole bag of chips or chug down one too many beers. It's damn near impossible to be blissful all the time, but even if the benefit of meditation is one less angry outburst, one more good night's sleep or one less headache, I'm sure you'll agree it's worth it.

If you're not exactly sure what meditation is, let me explain. You sit comfortably, close your eyes, and pay attention to your breathing. Feel the air as it rushes in through your nose, fills your lungs from top to bottom and then empties back out again. Repeat. You'll naturally start to breathe more slowly and deeply. Notice what thoughts come into your head—like what you want for dinner, or whether you should ask for a raise at work—no matter what it is, label it as a 'thought', then redirect your attention to your breath. When you catch yourself daydreaming, planning, analysing or worrying (which will happen constantly), just let the thoughts float away and refocus on the air flowing through your body. Keep doing this for 10–15 minutes and then gently return your attention to the room you're in.

NinjaMove

GET YOUR ZEN ON
Breathe in. Exhale all the way out. Hold for a few seconds without breathing in or out. Allow the breath to return. Continue to allow the body to breathe without effort. Let the body resume its natural breathing rhythm, so you are a witness to the breath instead of a participant in it. In your mind, watch the 'in' breath and the 'out' breath, taking note of the inhales and exhales. Let it do whatever it does ... If you can master this simple technique you will be amazed by how quickly you become relaxed, clear and present, more at ease and happier.

STRETCH YOUR POWER

Heel-to-toe warrior walks—Targets: core and leg muscles
Imagine you are walking on a tightrope. Extend your arms out to the sides and place one foot directly in front of the other for twenty steps.

Warrior clock cycles—Targets: quadriceps and core
Stand with your hands on your hips. Imagine that you are standing in the centre of a clock. Stand on your right leg, knee bent and extend your left leg out in front of you with your foot lightly touching the ground. One by one, touch your foot to every hour on the left side of the clock. Then change legs. Repeat four times.

Ninja leg lifts—Targets: glutes and the surrounding hip joints
Stand with your legs shoulder-width apart and hands on hips. Shift your weight over your right leg, then slowly swing your left leg behind you, lifting it as far off the ground as you can. Keep your right foot planted firmly on the ground with the knee slightly bent. Hold for a few seconds. Repeat ten to fifteen times.

Among the latest and most mind-blowing research on meditation is the discovery that it affects your brain the way exercise affects your body—making it stronger, healthier and more efficient. Experienced meditators produce more gamma brain waves, which are associated with intense, clear thinking and heightened cooperation between various parts of the brain. If brain waves were petrol, gammas would be the ultra-premium stuff. And the best thing? Just like the way the positive changes from exercise persist once you stop, these mega-meditators' brains had been trained to work better around the clock.

What's more, it looks like regular meditation may wind back and prevent the effects of ageing on the brain. Just as the brain part in charge of motor skills is more developed in athletes, the area of the brain that deals with attention and sensory perception is more developed in meditators. So meditating can stave off the brain fuzzies long-term. And right now, you might like to know that 40 minutes of meditation might perk you up more than a 40-minute nap. And let's not forget meditation's hightest claim: RELAXATION IS SO RELAXING.

I meditate for a few minutes every day, for inner peace, yes, but also to strengthen my confidence and presence of mind so I can focus on my dreams and put the stress of daily life in perspective. At the end of a rough day, meditation takes the edge off faster than any cocktail could. Yeah, it's that good.

KITCHEN KUNG FU

Being a weightloss warrior is all about training—and that includes our palates. We don't need to slather our meals with sauces if we're eating naked. If you think you might be overdoing the squirts, check your dirty dishes. Are there more spoons than knives and forks? It takes a fork to dig into healthier stuff like crisp salads, vegetables and chewy lean meats.

Pay yourself a condiment. Stick to low-calorie, low-sodium versions of your favourite squirts. Balsamic spray, low-salt tomato paste/sauce, low-salt soy sauce, salsa, horseradish, chilli sauce and lemon are warrior winners.

Bin reduced-fat, sugar-free, fat-free, low-carb products and eat naked instead. Flavour your meal with antioxidant-rich spices like cumin, dill, garlic, ginger, mint, parsley, rosemary, thyme. Get the pure form—cinnamon rather than cinnamon-sugar. Reduce the sugar in cake and biscuit recipes gradually until you've decreased it by one-third or more. Use equal amounts of unsweetened apple puree in place of oil or sugar. Add fat friends to baking and cereals in the form of nuts like almond flakes, pine nuts and walnuts.

Bake, barbeque, boil, braise, broil, roast, poach, steam or dry sauté food instead of frying.

You are allowed treats. I love treats! Just remember, don't eat anything your Nanna wouldn't recognise!

THE HAPPY WARRIOR

Happiness comes from deeds as well as words. Weightloss warriors need to apply positivity to all their actions. Here's how:

Happy swallows
Rather than labelling food as 'healthy' or 'junk', just eat naked and think of food as fuel for your body, which will give you different amounts of energy. This simple shift in perception can help you make better food choices.

Happy halves
Going absolutely cold turkey on everything is a major challenge. So take your worst food habit (say, pizza twice a week) and halve it (pizza once a week). You'll lose weight straight away.

Happy-tude
Dump the all-or-nothing attitude that manifests in thoughts like 'I've already eaten one doughnut, might as well eat the last five'. Remind yourself that one binge alone will never make you gain weight. It's what you do afterwards that matters. We all have weak moments where we lapse into our old habits. But what's important is that you recognise the destructive habit, stop and then renew your pledge to honour your mind, body and sprit with good choices.

Happy focus
When you're bored, instead of heading on autopilot straight to the nearest bickie jar, change your focus and get out of the house. It doesn't have to be about exercising or being productive, just do something you'll enjoy: go window-shopping or head to the movies. When you change your focus you change the way you feel, when you change the way you feel, you will change your appetite. You might find that you're not hungering for food, but stimulation, relaxation or connection.

Happy goals
The word 'should', with its overtones of authority, is de-motivating because it makes you feel something is lacking. Instead, give yourself a concrete goal. Say, 'I'm going to check out that pump class tomorrow,' instead of 'I should exercise more'.

Happy karma
Beat stress with this daily calming technique: sit in a quiet, comfortable place. Take slow, deep breaths and repeat the word 'power' to yourself as you exhale, for 2–3 minutes.

Happy brain
If you catch yourself thinking, 'I'll never lose weight,' stop what you're doing—I mean literally stand still. Then replace that negative thought with a positive one like: 'Okay, my body isn't as lean and fit as I'd like, but I'm making progress'. Weightloss warriors train the brain to discipline the body.

Tiff's Tip
Don't be a TeleChubby. If you have a habit of eating in front of the TV, keep your hands busy instead of your mouth— paint your nails or better yet get busy and do some stretches.

NinjaMove
ROCK'N'ROLL MASSEUSE
I don't mean to sound weird, but the best masseuse I've ever found is my tennis ball. Sit on the floor with your feet out in front of you and put the ball under your leg to massage deep into your hamstring and glutes. Roll it under your calf or lie down and roll it across your shoulders and middle back. If you can't get a foot rub from your partner, try rolling a golf ball under the soles of your feet. It feels amazing!

The posed warrior

We've been talking the whole way through this book about all the ways we can draw power from behaving like warriors in every area of weight loss. So now we're going to, quite literally, stand like warriors by learning 'warrior pose'. This comes from yoga, which is a physical practice that keeps you in your heart. It's about connecting with yourself, which is what you need most when you're healing, growing and changing. Yoga, with its heart-opening postures that release tightness in your chest, can actually make your heart feel lighter, brighter and more receptive to the love coming from friends and family around you. Your appetite and energy are strongly connected to your sense of self, or self-awareness. When you come to understand your body's needs more intimately, the perseverance you need to remain at your fighting weight will come more easily, as will the ability to self-nurture.

Warrior pose 1

1. Begin standing tall with your feet together and arms by your sides.
2. Step your legs about 1 metre apart, keeping your feet parallel. Inhale and lift your arms overhead, shoulder-width apart, palms facing each other.
3. Exhale and turn your left foot and leg 90 degrees out to the left and your right foot in 45 degrees to the left. Rotate your hips and torso to face the direction of your left leg.
4. Take a deep breath and as you exhale, bend your left knee, forming a right angle with your left thigh and shin. Hold for three to ten slow, deep breaths.

 (Tips: Less than 90 degrees is fine; only bend your front knee as far as you can, while keeping the outer edge of your back foot pressing flat into the floor, to stabilise the pose. Pull up through the arch of your back foot to avoid collapsing this ankle. To align your spine, draw your front ribs in, point your tailbone toward the floor and elongate the back of your neck, gazing straight ahead.)

Tiff's Tip

Repeat this mantra while inhaling: 'I am a weightloss warrior,' and while exhaling: 'Strong, powerful and centred'.

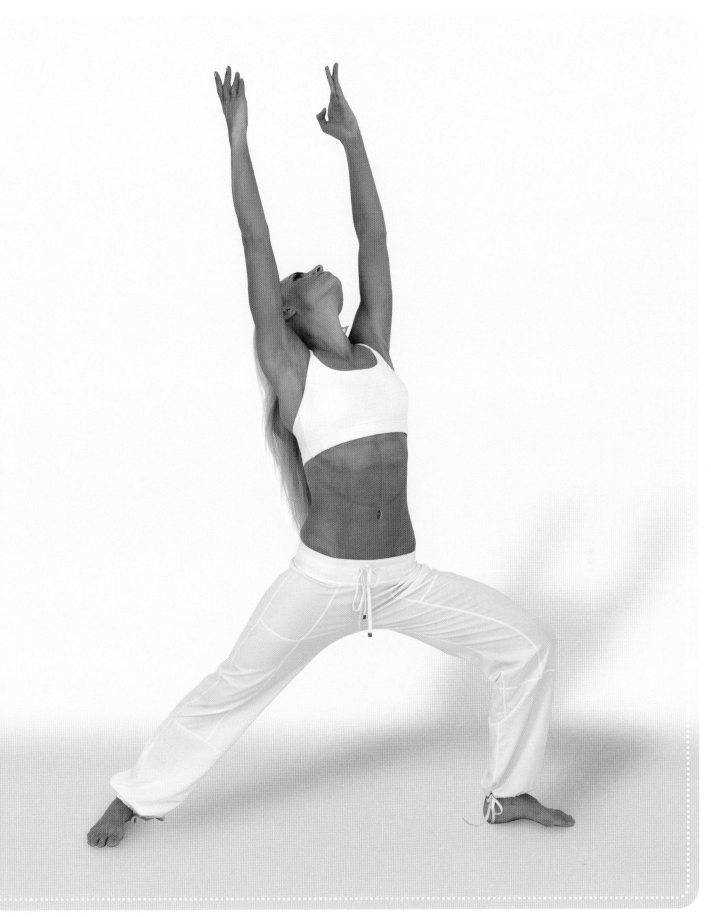

Warrior pose 2

1. Stand with feet parallel and hip-width apart.
2. Keeping your left leg strong, place the sole of your right foot against your inner left thigh.
3. Hug the muscles of your legs to the bones and push the right foot and left thigh together.
4. Bring your hands together in prayer position.

Repeat this mantra on the inhale: 'Balance is strength. When I love my body, my body loves me back,' and on the exhale: 'Health is beauty. Balance is power'.

Swaying back and forth? It's okay, trees sway in the wind too. The focus of this pose teaches you to channel your energy away from your emotional turmoil and into the task at hand: balance. The more secure you begin to feel in this pose, the more secure you will feel emotionally too.

HEALTHY NINJA HABITS

When you're tired, stressed or busy, old habits and old excuses can creep back in. One dessert here, a drive-through meal there, a week slips by without exercise … and before you know it your pants are feeling tight again and you'd rather keep up with the Kardashians on TV than keep up with the treadmill. Refresh what you've learnt since white belt with these 'stay naked forever' food swaps.

SWAP	FOR
Always eating birthday cake	Occasionally eating birthday cake (someone is always going to be having a birthday in the office)
Eating in bed	Reading or doing a puzzle—keep your mind and hands busy and away from food
Eating your whole meal	Saving some for lunch tomorrow
Fattening sauces	Homemade salsa
Weighing yourself every day	Weighing your food every day—soon you'll be able to eyeball the correct portion size
Eating in front of the TV	Stretching in front of the TV
A last-minute menu choice	A planned meal
Egg yolks	Eggwhites, or swap eggs altogether for hummus
Two pieces of bread	One piece of bread—instead of eating a sandwich with top and bottom try making a version of your favourite without a lid
Mayo	Avocado
Sugar	Sweet spice—add nutmeg or cinnamon to smoothies, cereal, yoghurt, tea or coffee (these also add powerful antioxidants)
White breadcrumbs and croutons	Wholemeal breadcrumbs and croutons

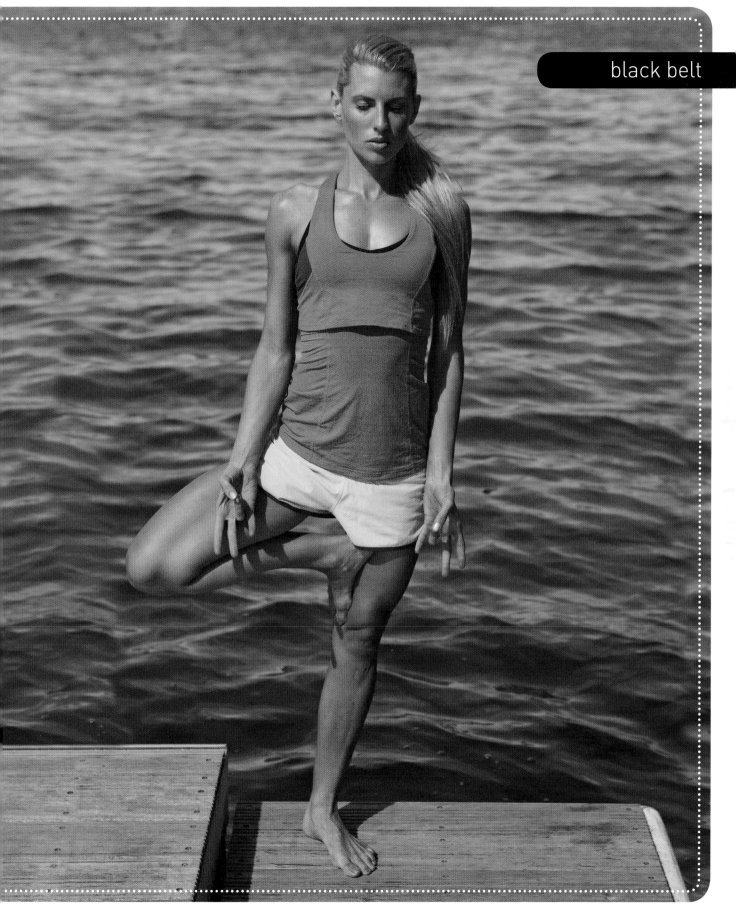

Resting pose (savasana)

Practise this pose whenever you have trouble relaxing or falling asleep. It will help you Zen out, because lying horizontally promotes calm and serenity, while the support of the floor and blankets makes you feel coddled.

1. You will need two beach towels or blankets. Roll one very tightly. Fold the second into a pillow.

2. Begin by lying on the floor and placing the rolled blanket horizontally beneath your shoulder blades (where your bra line is, for the ladies).

3. Rest your head on the second blanket, making sure that your heart is higher than your head.

4. Close your eyes and stay here breathing deeply for 2–5 minutes, focusing on releasing your upper body down into the blankets.

5. Let go of whatever emotions may have bubbled up during your practice. Let go of the tension you're holding in your body.

Repeat the mantra: 'I am in the now. I create my thoughts and my thoughts create my life'.

Warriors are prepared

Now I'm not saying that restaurant or fast food is okay for everyday eating, but the weightloss warrior has to be flexible and able to defend themselves when eating out. You might get ensnared by the golden arches and held hostage by your little ninjas, and you don't want to feel awkward or sabotaged when socialising. So for special occasions, when you and your tribe are out with friends, or on the interstate highway with no nude food to be found, remember your ninja moves and you will sail through unscathed and stay motivated.

Fast-food moves

Avoid all upsized meals or anything with the words 'super,' 'triple' or 'whopper'. Opt for smaller portions, or share larger portions. Ignore meal deals—go a side salad, corn cob or yoghurt instead. Avoid butter and margarine when ordering sandwiches to rescue 100 calories (418 kJ). Never eat a fast-food dessert.

Here are the keys to navigating the main chains:

At Burger King: ask for the Veggie Whopper. This includes all the trimmings minus the meat patty. Rescues 240 calories (1,004 kJ).

At Grill'd (and other gourmet burger joints): ask for sandwiches 'protein style' (to get a lettuce leaf instead of a bun), or a 'bun-less burger' to rescue 70 calories (293 kJ). Or hold the meat on your cheeseburger to rescue 100 calories (418 kJ).

At Mexican joints: ask for burrito 'streaker style' and they'll drop the tortilla to rescue 310 calories (1,297 kJ). Or ask for any burrito on the menu to 'go naked' and it will arrive without the standard tortilla. Also works for salads served in a taco shell. Rescue 300 calories (1,255 kJ).

At Starbucks: order short size and they'll shrink your drink to an eight-ounce cup. Rescues 140–350 calories (586-1,465 kJ).

At Boostjuice: choose low-fat smoothies or a crush over a fruit juice. Lowest calorie smoothies (original size) are Skinnie Minnie Melon (280 calories (1,172 kJ)), Energy Life (416 calories (1,741 kJ)) and All Berry Bang (377 calories (1,578 kJ)). Always opt for berries–the lowest calorie fruit. Add protein powder to any drink. For 30 calories (125 kJ) you'll add 6 grams of protein and 1 gram of fibre to fill you up. Remember these drinks are meals.

At Subway: order any sandwich as a salad to rescue up to 520 calories (2,176 kJ). Although Subway markets its '6 grams of fat or less' sandwiches as healthy options, if you add cheese, mayonnaise or some other sauces the fat content will skyrocket to equal a Macca's meal. Also stick with a 6-inch, not a foot-long.

At McDonald's: The Lighter Choices or Heart Foundation Tick range are okay but be wary of the M selections as some foods have the same calorie count as a Big Mac.

At Red Rooster: go the skin-free chicken range most of which have less than 10 grams of fat. Never go near the Ripper Sub rolls with more than 20 grams of fat per individual serve. No shanks!

At Pizza Hut: order any pizza 'fit'n'delicious' style to get half the cheese and extra sauce and vegies. Save 400 calories (1,674 kJ) for a personal pizza, 100–300 calories (418-1,255 kJ) per slice of a medium pizza. The healthiest option is the thin'n'crispy vegetarian pizza. Salami is the worst.

NinjaNewsflash

WORK *HARD* AND LONG
When you exercise at a higher intensity you get fitter, your aerobic energy system works more efficiently and you burn more fat 24 hours a day, 7 days a week. Harder workouts will burn more calories overall, because of their greater energy cost. Most people can exercise either hard or long— weightloss warriors aim for both. SO GET YA NINJA ON!

WHEN TO SWEAT IT OUT

FIGHT ON IF ...

You have a mild cold—back off to 60 per cent. Exercising at this level won't exacerbate your illness but will maintain your conditioning.

You have a headache—exercise will boost the chemicals you need to release the tight pressure in your head.

You're hungover—exercise will help mobilise the toxins from the alcohol. Keep hydration up because alcohol has already dehydrated you.

You're feeling down—regular exercise increases the brain's levels of serotonin, a neuro-transmitter involved in mood, sleep, appetite and other issues linked with depression.

BOW OUT IF ...

You have a fever—exercise will make your temperature rise more, which can put your heart under strain. Rest.

You have aches and pains—body aches are often the first sign of the flu or a more serious virus. Back off—the sore muscles can put you at greater risk of injury.

You have breathing problems—avoid exercising in cold, dry air. If you have asthma, take your medication and wait 4 minutes, then get back into it only if symptoms disappear.

Your stomach is upset or you have diarrhoea or are vomiting—avoid strenuous activity.

You have a heavy cough—anything that affects your airways is not good.

EAT NAKED FOR LIFE

Treat meat as a garnish and eat vegies and salads with abandon. Find a way to eat vegies for breakfast, lunch and dinner. They supply most nutrients and are extra-low in calories. The exception is starchier vegies like pumpkin and sweet potato, which are higher in calories and carbs, so one serving a day is plenty.

Go for weed. Seaweed! The fibre in seaweed reduces the amount of fat absorbed in the body by up to 75 per cent.

Trade rice every now and then for lentils to kick up your protein and fibre levels. Half a cup of lentils has 10 grams of protein.

Exchange traditional yoghurt for Greek-style yoghurt. It has the same calories per cup but twice the protein and half the carbs. Its velvety texture makes a great base for dips too.

If you can't cook—go frozen. But always check the sodium content and avoid frozen foods in syrups or packed with sugar.

Eat one raw vegie a day—keeping sliced vegies in the fridge for snacking makes this easy. Try capsicum, celery and carrot.

Each week eat from the Vegie Rainbow. Choosing fruits and vegies from the six key colour groups—red, orange, yellow, light green, dark green and purple—ensures a variety of nutrients in your diet.

Avoid dried fruits: raisins, sultanas, dried apricots. They are often treated with additives, overly concentrated in calories and fruit sugar—havoc for hormones. Five dried apricots equates to 3 teaspoons of M&M's.

Always choose whole fruits over fruit juices. Fruit juices have no fibre and therefore do little to help you control your appetite or make you feel full.

Always opt for cooking oil spray to minimise added fat and use a little, not a lot. If you like to use a particular cooking oil—buy a spray bottle and fill it with your healthy cooking oil of choice. Olive, avocado and walnut oils are good choices.

Peanut butter: low-sodium, reduced-fat peanut butter is best.

Try other nut spreads (cashew, almond) with celery sticks or carrots.

Tap into unhulled tahini.

Avoid the squirts. Be aware of sauces, toppings, dressings, spreads—these are empty calories, salt-packed and can double or triple your meal caloric intake as well as dull your taste buds.

Decode the menu

Weightloss warriors don't need to feel under attack when they go out for dinner. You just need a few moves up your sleeve to help you steer clear of restaurant food traps.

Look for these safe houses: baked, barbequed, boiled, braised, broiled, broth, coulis, garden-fresh, grilled, poached, raw, roasted, salsa, steamed. Be aware of and avoid high-fat code words: aioli, alfredo, au gratin, bacon, battered, bechamel, beurre, bisque, breaded, buttered, carbonara, casserole, cheesy, club, creamed, creamy, crispy, crumbed, crunchy, crusted, curry, deep-fried, fried, fritter, golden brown, old-fashioned, meaty, rich, sautéed, smothered, stuffed, tempura, the works, ultimate.

Eat a healthy snack before a late dinner so you don't arrive starving and hoe in to the bread basket. In fact, ask the waiter NOT to bring out the bread basket at all.

Skip soft drink and alcohol.

Order first. You will be less influenced by other people's choices. Order two entrées, order a main meal entrée size or share a main with a friend if there are no healthy main options. Ask for salad with all sauces and dressings to be served on the side.

Make special requests:

'Hold the … (cheese, cream, sour cream, chicken skin, butter, margarine, mayonnaise).'

'Can you please use minimal … (oil, butter, cheese, salad dressing?)'

'Could you add more … vegetables, salad?'

'May I substitute this ingredient for … (sliced tomatoes, salad, fresh fruit, lemon, balsamic vinegar?)'

Dodge dessert danger by ordering a fresh fruit salad, a cappuccino instead, un-iced cake, herbal tea, fruit sorbet, or order one dessert to share.

Stride on warriors

This journey is never over—it lasts your whole life and drives you to reach and expand your full potential. When you achieve a centred happiness in yourself, and a genuine connection with your body, your mind, your tribe, your environment and your dreams, that is the sign of true health. Only then can we really know and honour ourselves.

Fully fledged warriors have found the passion that brings them alive. You will recognise your passion when something inspires energy, excitement and the feeling that the world is opening up around you. That is when you're the most powerful warrior you can be. That is when you've truly earned your black belt in health. When you recognise, accept and embrace your true nature, and live joyfully in the here and now, you will stride forward into your future, armed with the warrior power, vitality and passion to not only remain inspired but also inspire others.

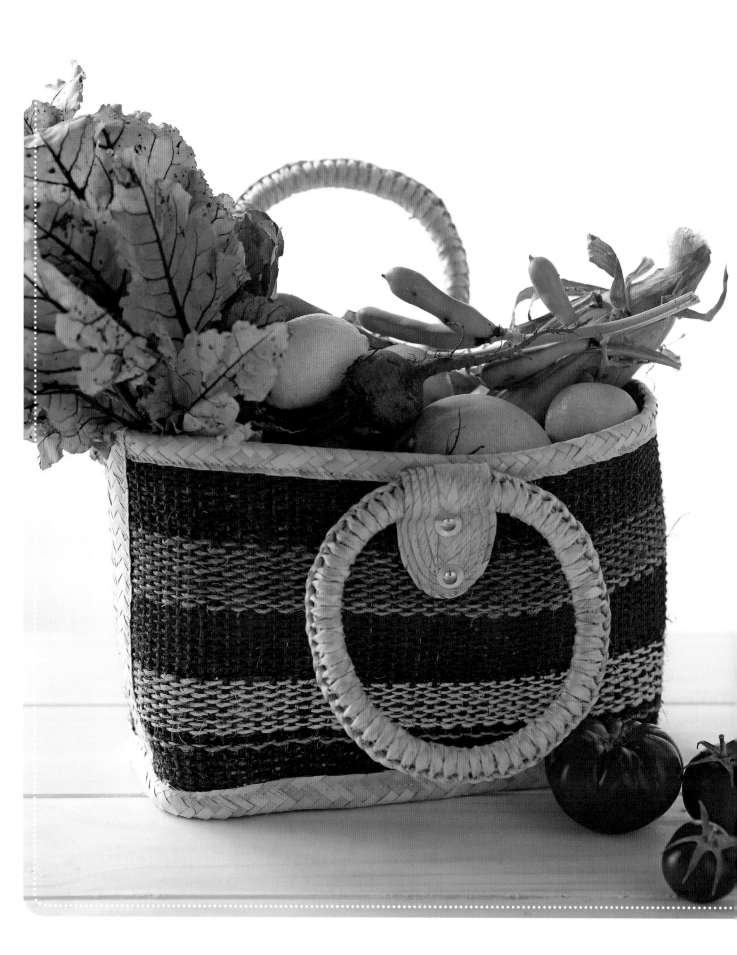

Warrior recipes

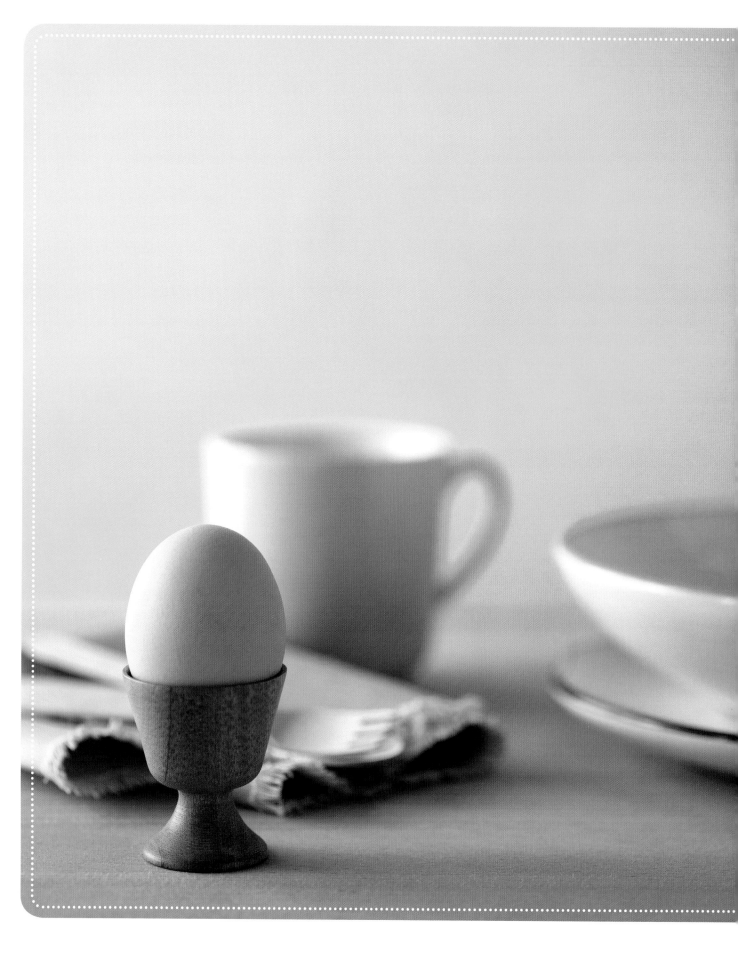

hearty breakfasts

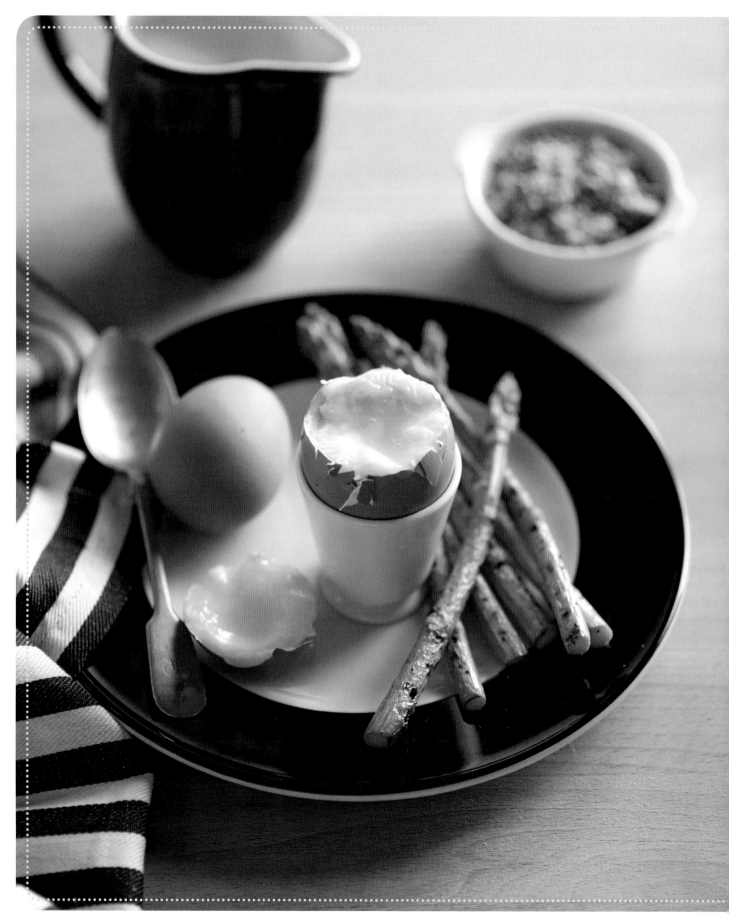

Soft-boiled eggs with grilled asparagus and dukkah

SERVES 1

DUKKAH

75 g (½ cup) sesame seeds

50 g (⅓ cup) hazelnuts

55 g (⅓ cup) almonds

30 g coriander seeds

30 g cumin seeds

salt to taste

To make the dukkah, toast all the seeds and nuts separately until fragrant, either in a dry frypan or on a baking tray in a preheated oven at 180°C.

Allow to cool, then combine and crush roughly in a mortar and pestle or pulse in a food processor until coarsely ground. Add salt to taste. Store the dukkah in an airtight container in a cool, dry place for up to six weeks.

2 eggs

200 g asparagus, trimmed

1 tablespoon extra—virgin olive oil

salt and freshly ground black pepper

Bring a large saucepan of water to the boil and gently lower the eggs into the water. Boil for 3–4 minutes, depending on how soft you like them.

To prepare the asparagus, toss with the oil, salt and pepper. Sauté in a grill pan over a medium–high heat for 4–5 minutes, turning occasionally until golden brown.

To serve, place the eggs into egg cups and crack the top. Dip the asparagus spears into the runny egg yolk and then into the dukkah.

Wholewheat blueberry pancakes

MAKES 16

200 g (1⅓ cups) wholewheat flour

1½ teaspoons baking powder

pinch of salt

1 egg

500 ml (2 cups) buttermilk

extra-virgin olive oil for cooking

150 g fresh blueberries

Combine the flour, baking powder and salt in a bowl. In a separate bowl, mix the egg and buttermilk. Pour the egg mixture into the flour and stir until smooth.

Heat half a teaspoon of oil in a heavy-based frying pan over a medium–high heat. Add a large spoonful (around 2 tablespoons) of the batter and swirl to coat the base of the pan, or until approximately 8 centimetres in diameter. Sprinkle three or four blueberries over the pancake and cook until bubbles start to form. Turn the pancake over and cook until golden brown, for approximately 2 minutes. Remove from the pan and cover with foil to keep warm.

Return the pan to the heat and repeat with remaining batter.

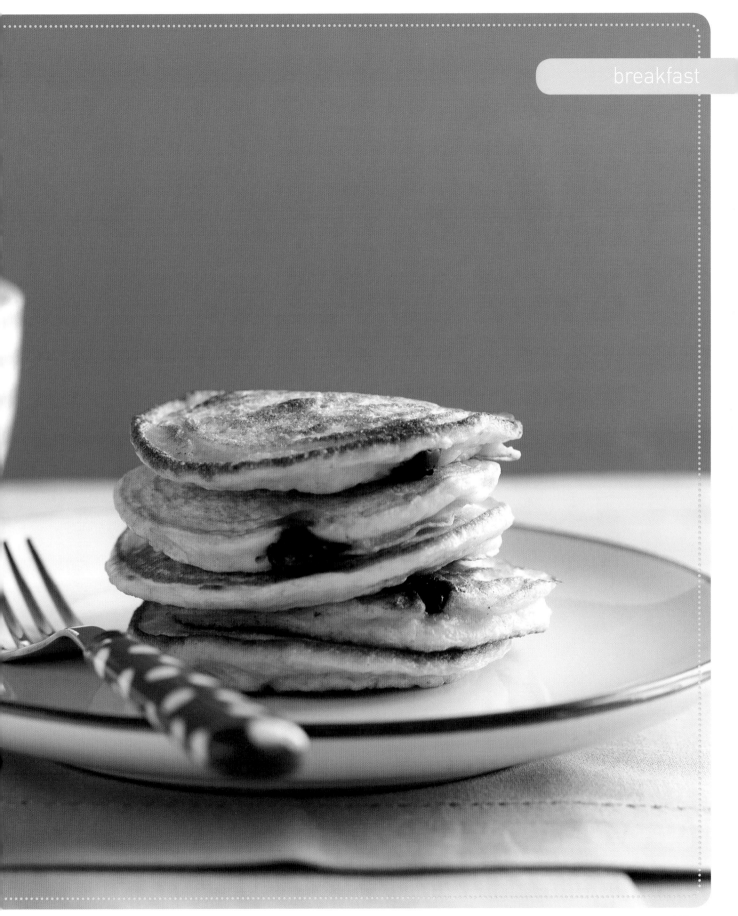

Eggwhite omelette with spinach, capsicum and mushroom

SERVES 1

1 teaspoon extra-virgin olive oil

½ red capsicum, finely sliced

100 g mushrooms, finely sliced

salt and freshly ground black pepper

50 g baby spinach

3 eggwhites

1 tablespoon flat-leaf parsley, chopped

Preheat oven to 180°C.

Heat half a teaspoon of olive oil in a 24-centimetre, ovenproof frying pan over a medium–high heat. Sauté the capsicum and mushrooms until soft, approximately 3–4 minutes. Season with salt and pepper. Add the spinach and cook until wilted, approximately 1 minute. Remove from the pan.

In a bowl, whisk the eggwhites until soft peaks form. Season with salt and freshly ground black pepper. Heat remaining oil in the pan over a medium heat, add the eggwhites and cook until nearly set, for about 2 minutes.

Sprinkle the vegetable filling over the omelette and top with the chopped parsley. Place the pan in the preheated oven and bake until the egg cooks through, approximately 3–4 minutes. Serve immediately.

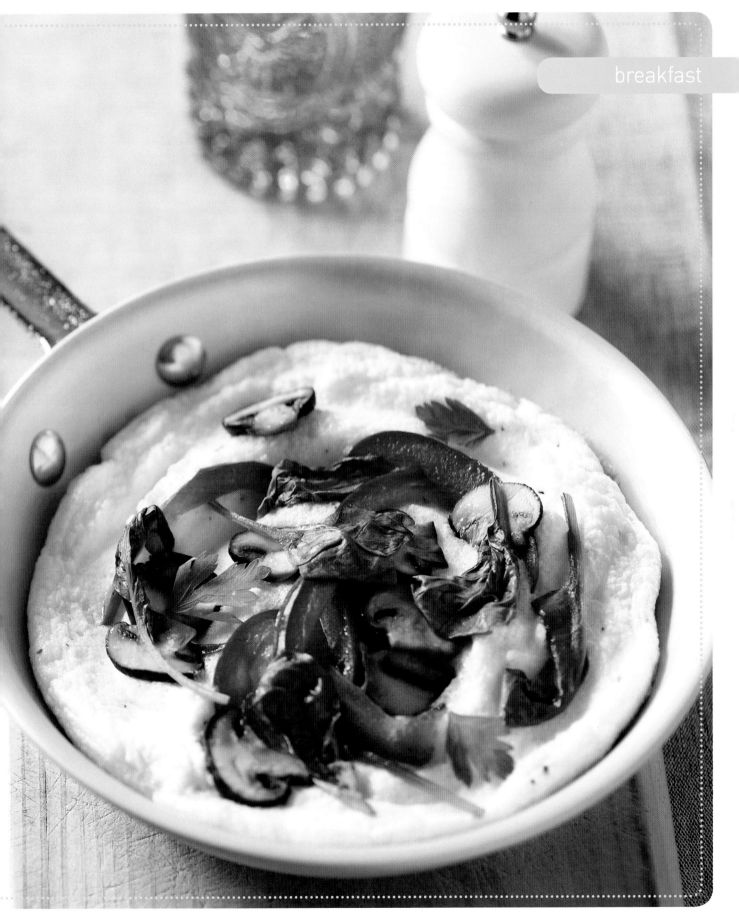

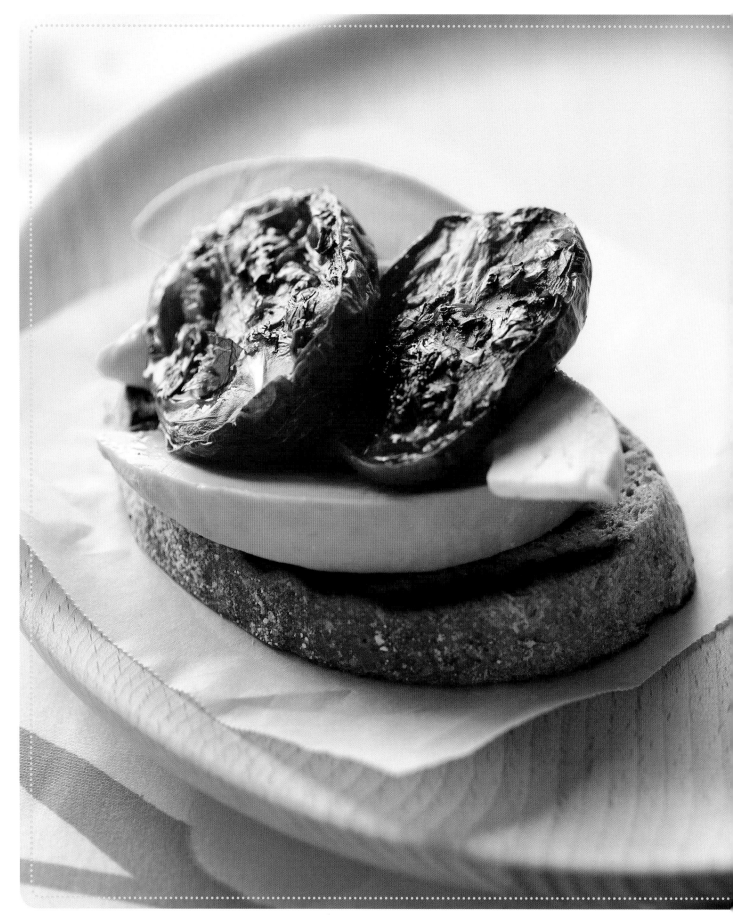

Avocado and roasted tomato on toast

SERVES 2

2 roma tomatoes

2 teaspoons of extra-virgin olive oil

2 tablespoons mixed herbs (such as parsley, basil and thyme), chopped

1 tablespoon balsamic vinegar

2 slices of bread (such as pumpernickel, dark rye or multigrain)

1 avocado, peeled and sliced

salt and freshly ground black pepper

Preheat oven to 180°C.

Cut the tomatoes in half and mix with the oil, salt, pepper, herbs and vinegar until evenly coated. Roast on a tray in the preheated oven for 30–40 minutes, or until tender.

Toast the bread until golden brown. Arrange two tomato halves and half an avocado each on piece of bread.

Cinnamon porridge with blueberries and honey

SERVES 2

100 g (1 cup) rolled oats

250 ml (1 cup) water

250 ml (1 cup) reduced-fat milk

½ teaspoon ground cinnamon

100 g fresh blueberries

honey for serving

Combine the oats, water, milk and cinnamon in a heavy-based saucepan. Bring to the boil, then reduce heat. Simmer, stirring occasionally, until porridge thickens and oats are cooked through, for 5–6 minutes.

Spoon porridge into bowls, scatter blueberries and drizzle honey over the top. Serve with extra milk if desired.

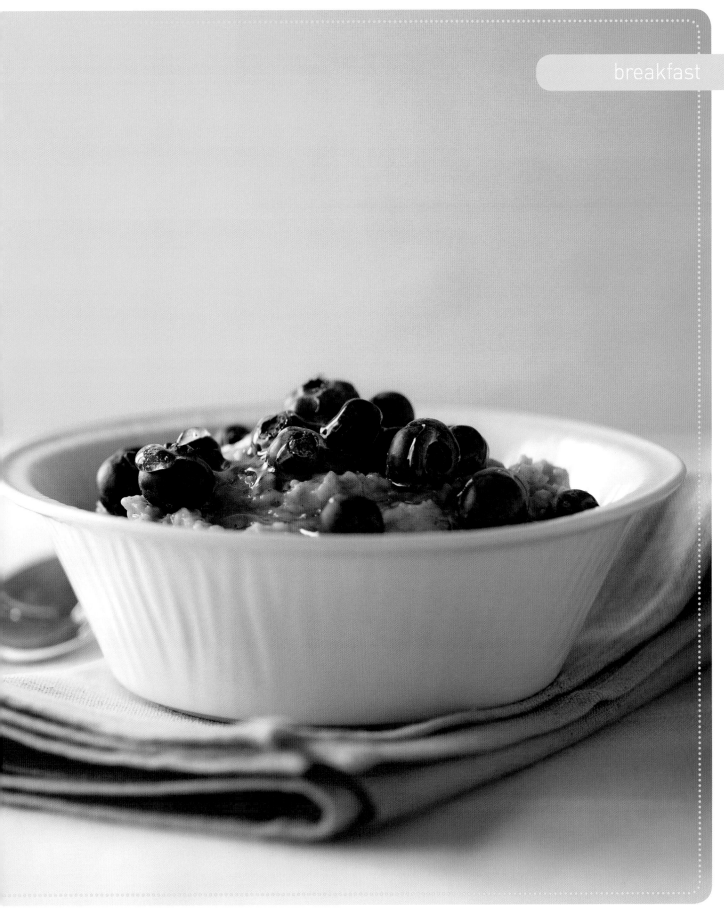

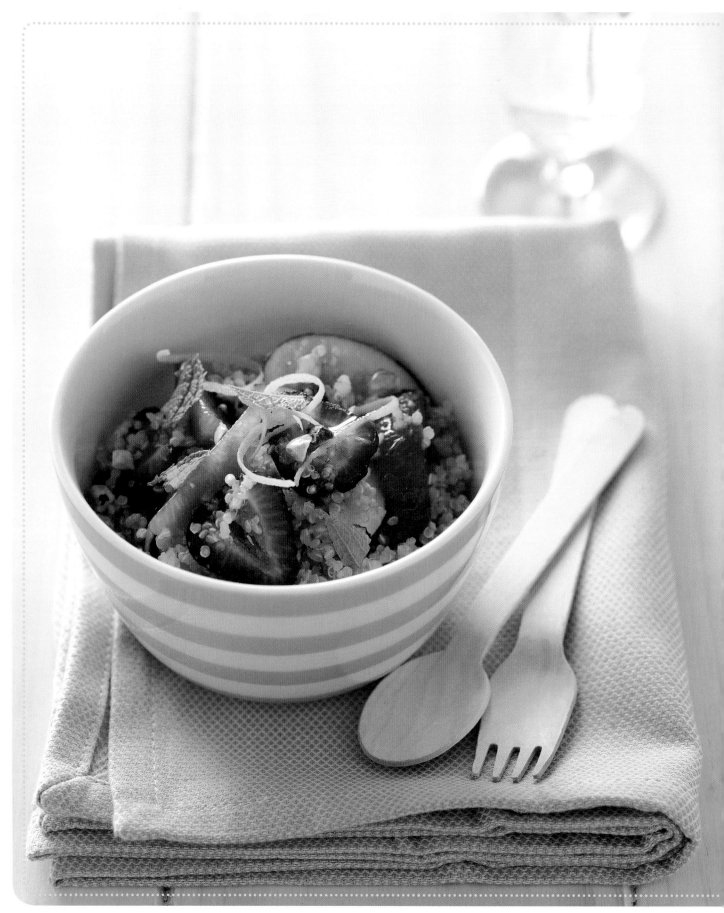

Breakfast quinoa with summer fruits

SERVES 4

100 g (1 cup) quinoa

zest of 1 orange

500 ml (2 cups) water

1 pink grapefruit

2 nectarines, sliced

250 g strawberries, washed and halved

4 mint leaves, finely sliced

75 g (½ cup) chopped pistachios, optional

honey to serve

Rinse quinoa in a small strainer. Combine with the orange zest and water in a small saucepan and bring to the boil. Reduce heat, cover and simmer for 10–12 minutes, until the water is absorbed and quinoa appears translucent.

While quinoa is cooking, peel the grapefruit with a sharp knife, removing the peel and outside pith. Cut down along the membranes to remove each segment. Mix grapefruit segments, nectarines, strawberries and chopped mint in a bowl and squeeze over any excess juice from the grapefruit pith.

Fluff the quinoa with a fork and divide between four bowls. Top with the fruit, pistachios and a drizzle of honey to serve.

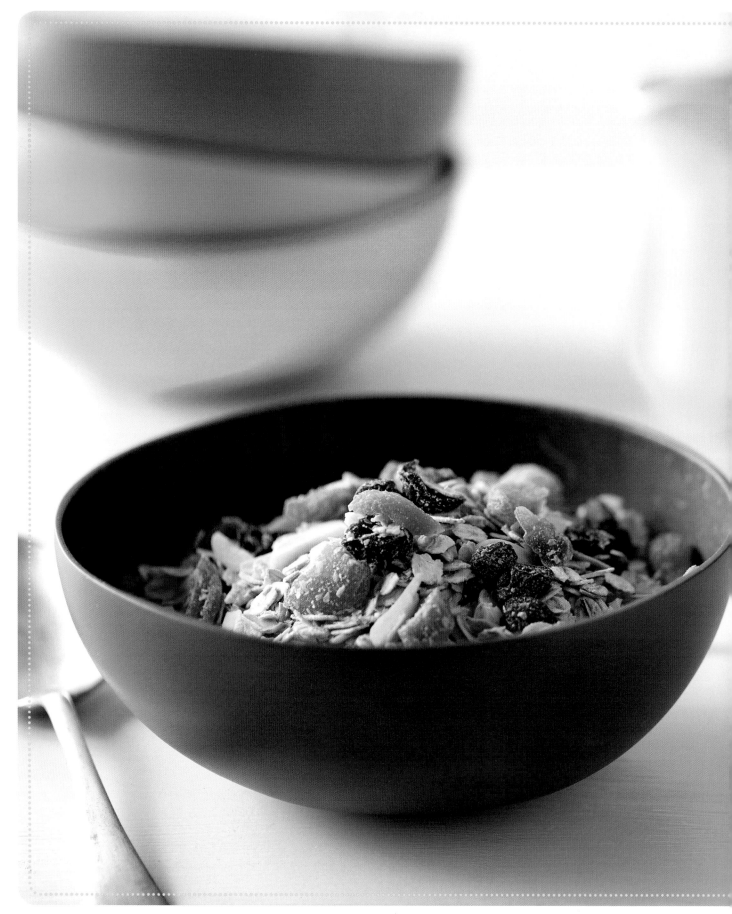

Almond and apricot muesli

MAKES APPROXIMATELY 10 CUPS

500 g (5 cups) rolled oats

90 g (½ cup) slivered almonds, toasted

150 g (1 cup) sultanas

150 g (1 cup) raisins

150 g (1 cup) dried apricots, chopped

60 g (1 cup) bran

80 g (½ cup) sunflower seeds or pumpkin seeds

Combine all ingredients. Store in an airtight container in a cool, dark place for up to 3 months.

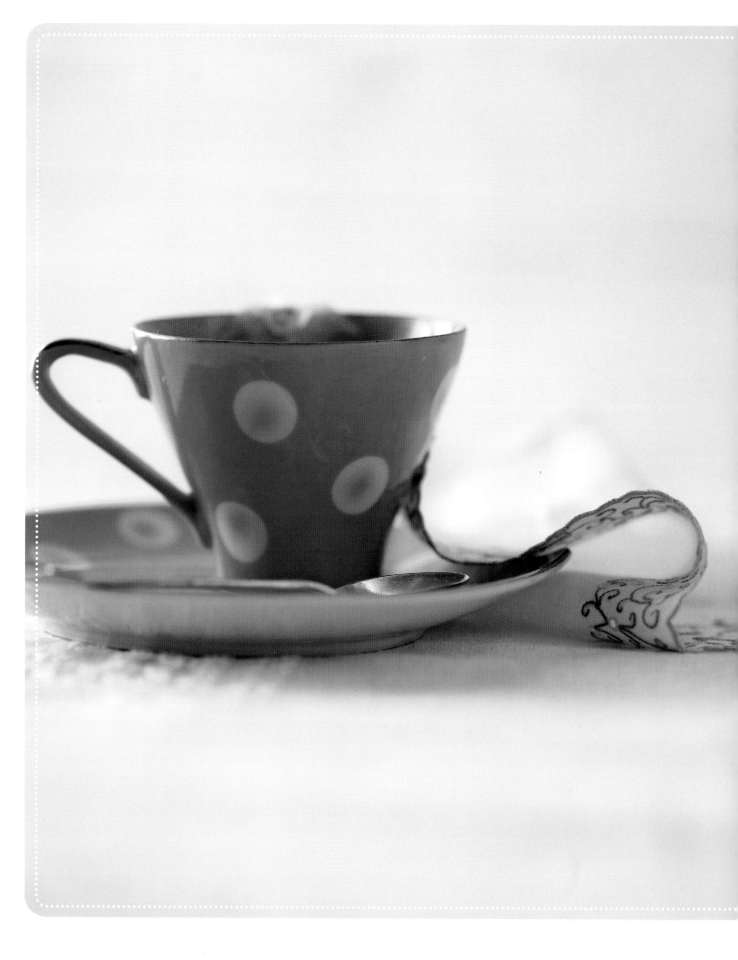

quick snacks

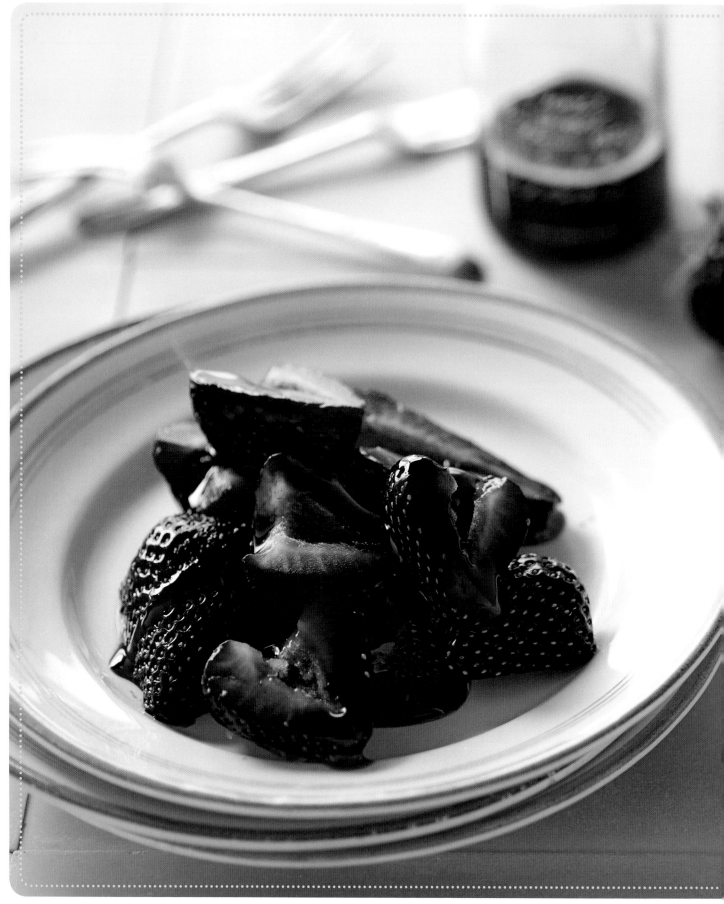

Strawberries with balsamic vinegar

SERVES 2

250 g (1 punnet) strawberries
1 tablespoon balsamic vinegar

Wash, hull and halve the strawberries.

Heat a small frying pan over a low heat and gently warm the balsamic vinegar until it reduces slightly and becomes viscous.

Pour the balsamic vinegar over the strawberries and toss to combine. Allow to stand at room temperature for 30 minutes.

Serve at room temperature for the best flavour. The brave can add a grind of fresh black pepper—delicious!

Fig and almond balls

MAKES 14

75 g (½ cup) dried figs

75 g (½ cup) dates

90 g (½ cup) chopped almonds

2 tablespoons tahini

2 tablespoons honey

2 teaspoons sesame seeds

45 g (½ cup) shredded coconut

Place all ingredients except for the coconut in a food processor and pulse until roughly combined.

Scoop out 1 tablespoon of mixture and, using damp hands, roll into a ball and dredge in coconut.

Repeat with remaining mixture.

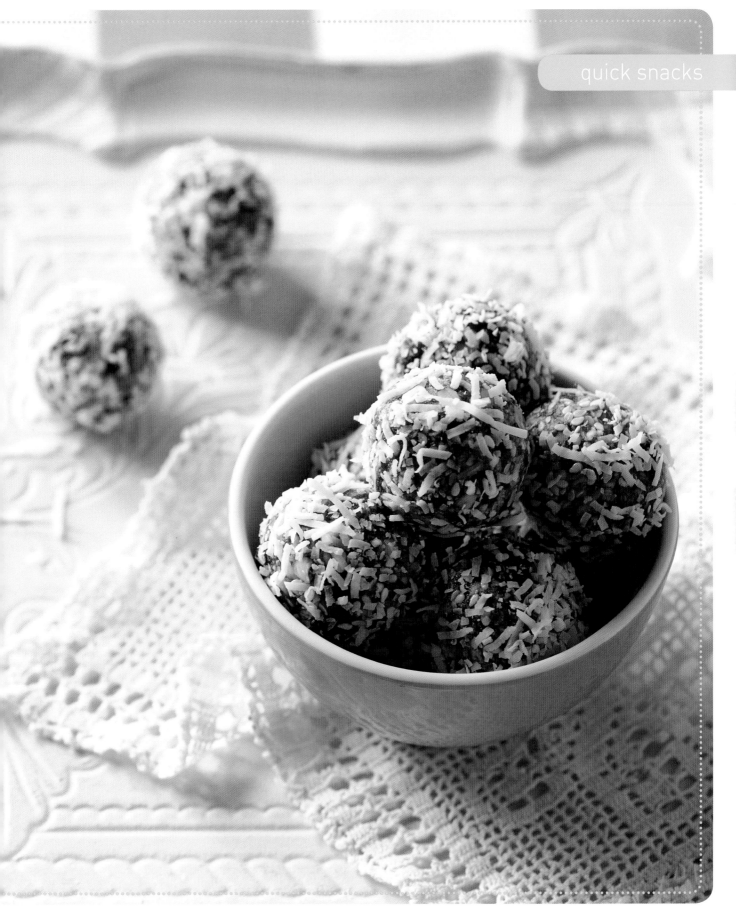

Muesli slice

MAKES 12

150 g (1 cup) self-raising flour

90 g (1 cup) shredded coconut

100 g (1 cup) rolled oats

75 g (½ cup) sultanas

75 g (½ cup) chopped dates

60 g (½ cup) sunflower seeds, optional

125 g butter

2 tablespoons water

80 g honey

1 egg

Preheat oven to 180°C.

Grease and line a 20 x 30 cm lamington tin.

Mix the flour, coconut, oats, dried fruit and seeds in a large bowl.

Melt the butter, water and honey in a saucepan over a low heat and pour over combined dry ingredients while still hot. Stir well until mixture comes together. Add the egg and combine well.

Spoon mixture into the lamington tin and bake in the preheated oven for 20 minutes, or until set and golden brown.

Allow to cool before cutting into wedges.

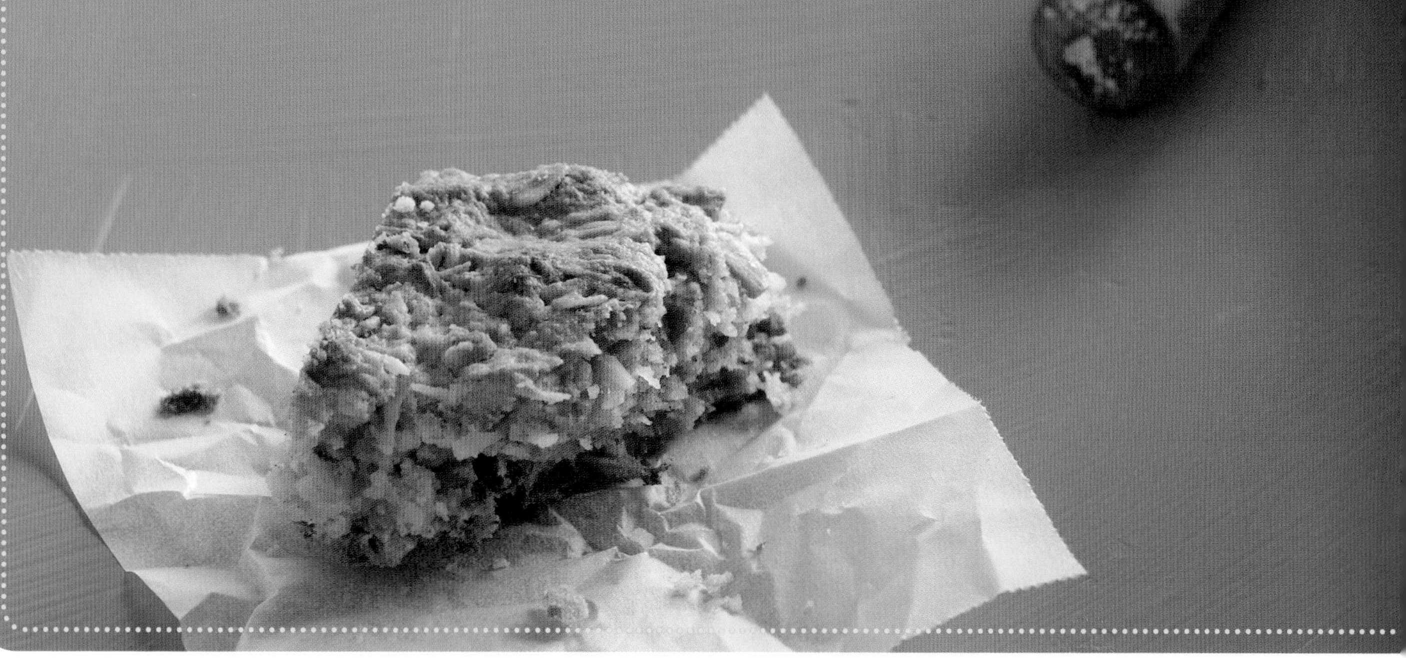

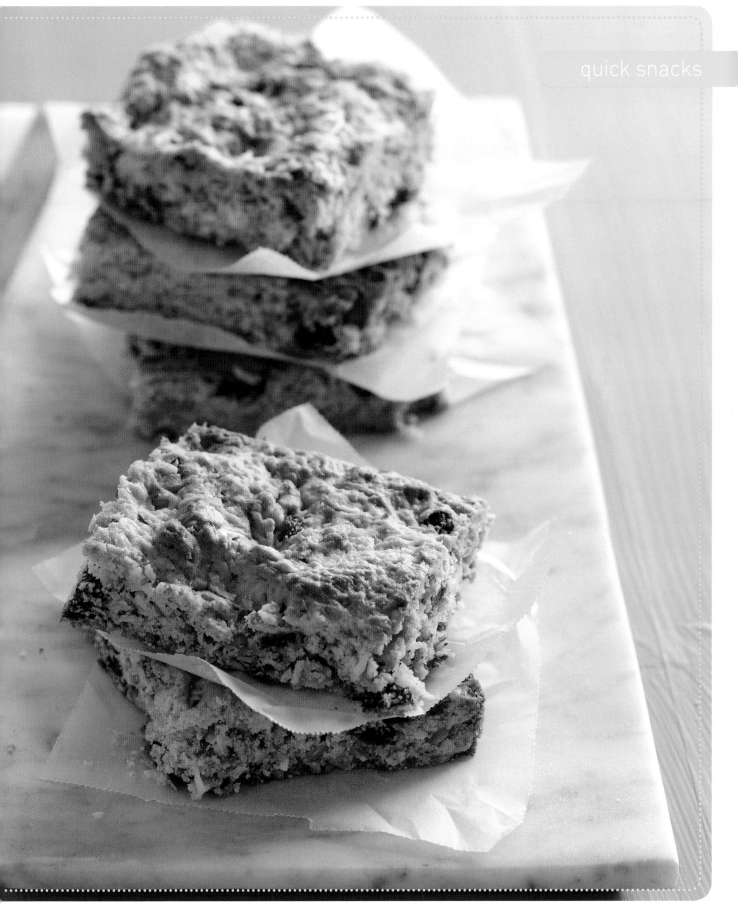

Hearty tabbouleh

SERVES 4

POMEGRANATE DRESSING
60 ml (¼ cup) extra-virgin olive oil
1 tablespoon lemon juice
1 tablespoon honey
2 teaspoons pomegranate molasses
salt and freshly ground black pepper

Combine all ingredients in a screwtop jar and shake well.

1 fresh pomegranate, optional
200 g (1 cup) burghul
1 red onion, finely sliced
1 cup flat-leaf parsley leaves
1 cup coriander leaves
120 g (1 cup) toasted walnuts, roughly chopped
400 g tin chickpeas, drained and rinsed

Soak the burghul in plenty of cold water for 30 minutes. Drain and tip into a large bowl.

If using the pomegrante, remove the seeds, discarding the bitter, yellow inside skin. Combine pomegranate with the burghul, reserving a tablespoon of the seeds. Add the onion, parsley, coriander, walnuts and chickpeas.

Toss with the dressing and garnish with the reserved pomegranate seeds just before serving. You can also boost the protein content by adding cooked lentils.

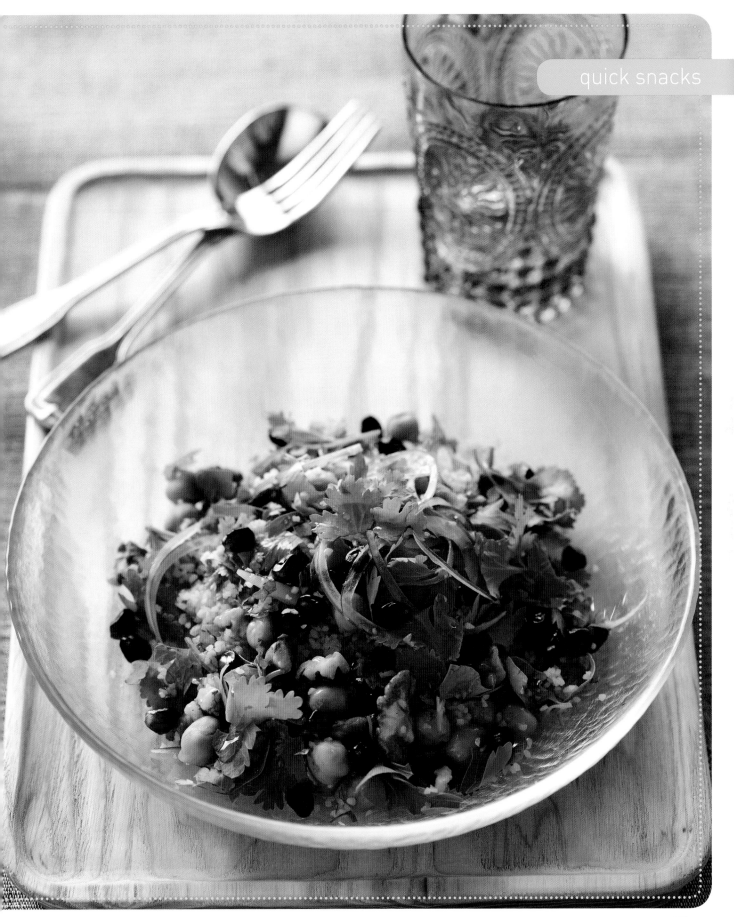

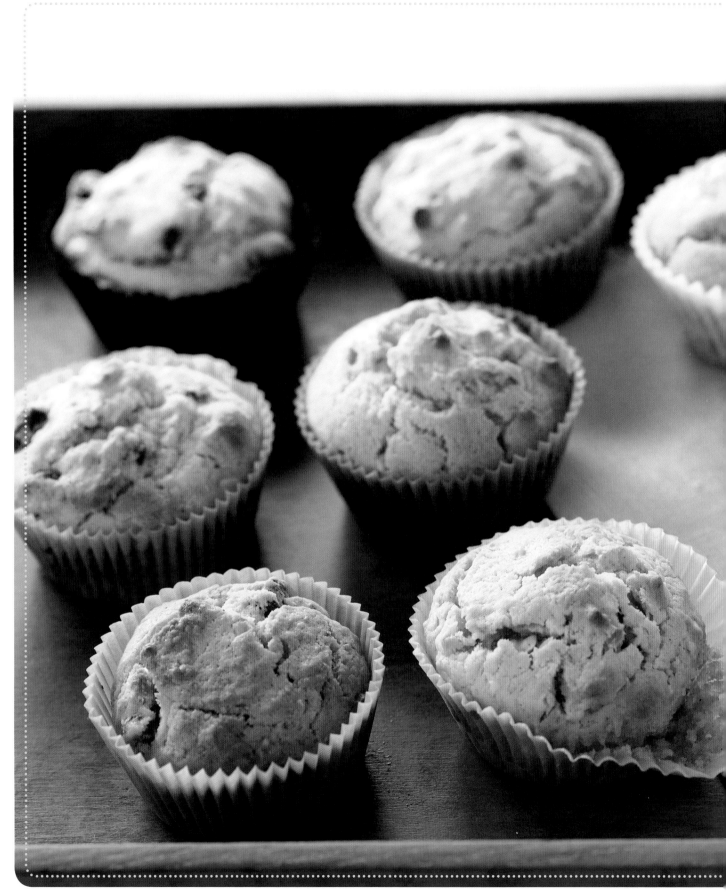

Pumpkin, cardamom and cashew muffins

MAKES 12

75 g (½ cup) sultanas

250 ml (1 cup) hot tea

170 g butter, softened

100 g honey

2 eggs

250 g (1⅔ cups) self-raising flour

250 g pumpkin, steamed
    or boiled and pureed

75 g (½ cup) cashews,
    roughly chopped

1 teaspoon ground cardamom

Preheat oven to 180°C. Grease a 12-hole muffin tin or line with patty cases.

Soak sultanas in hot tea for 15 minutes, drain well and discard tea.
Set sultanas aside.

Cream butter and honey until light and fluffy. Add eggs one by one, beating
well after each addition. Add flour and pumpkin puree, beat well. Stir in
sultanas, cashews and cardamom.

Pour into muffins tins and bake in the preheated oven for 15–18 minutes,
until risen and golden brown.

Roasted carrot hummus with fresh tomato salsa

SERVES 4, WITH PLENTY OF EXTRA HUMMUS

FRESH TOMATO SALSA

1 punnet cherry tomatoes, quartered

¼ cup flat-leaf parsley

¼ cup coriander leaves

1 tablespoon mint, chopped

2 tablespoons extra-virgin olive oil

1 tablespoon lemon juice

salt and freshly ground black pepper

Toss all ingredients until well combined.

3 carrots, peeled and diced

½ tablespoon extra-virgin olive oil

salt and freshly ground black pepper

400 g tin chickpeas, drained and rinsed

2 garlic cloves

2 tablespoons tahini

2 tablespoons lemon juice

60 ml (¼ cup) olive oil

1 teaspoon ground cumin

pumpernickel bread to serve

Preheat oven to 180°C.

Toss carrots with oil and a sprinkle of salt and pepper. Roast on a tray in the preheated oven for 20 minutes, or until tender.

Blend chickpeas and roasted carrot in a food processor until smooth. Add garlic, tahini, lemon juice, olive oil and cumin and blend again until all ingredients are smooth and well combined. Add extra salt and pepper and lemon juice if required.

To serve, spread a thick layer of the carrot hummus over sliced pumpernickel bread and top with tomato salsa.

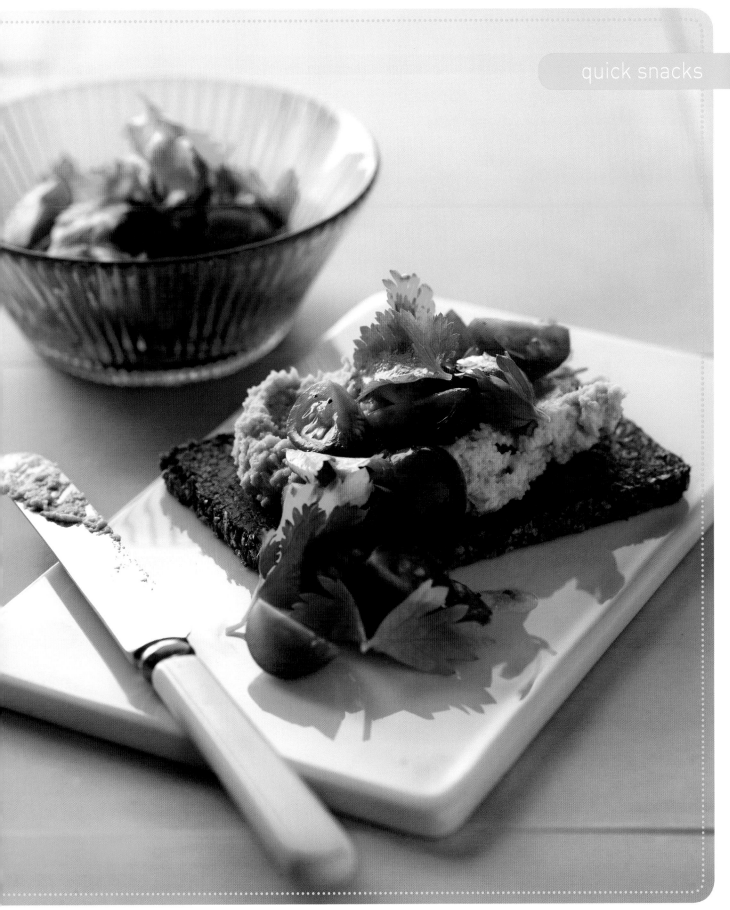

Fruity oat slice

MAKES 16 PIECES

240 g (1 ⅔ cups) mixed dried fruit (for example,
  apricots, figs, pears, peaches and apple),
  roughly chopped

150 g (1 cup) sultanas

440 g can crushed pineapple in natural juice

150 g butter

1 teaspoon mixed spice

½ teaspoon ground ginger

½ teaspoon cinnamon

2 eggs

100 g (⅔ cup) self-raising flour

150 g (1½ cups) rolled oats

8 dried apple rings

1 tablespoon honey

Preheat oven to 170°C.

Grease and line a 20 x 30 cm lamington tin.

Place the dried fruit, pineapple and juice, butter
and spices in a large saucepan over a low heat
until the butter melts. Allow to cool.

Add the eggs to the cooled fruit mixture and
stir well. Add the flour and oats and mix until
combined.

Spoon the mixture into the tin and decorate
with additional dried apple rings brushed with
a tablespoon of warmed honey. Bake in the
preheated oven for 20 minutes. Allow to cool
and cut into squares or fingers.

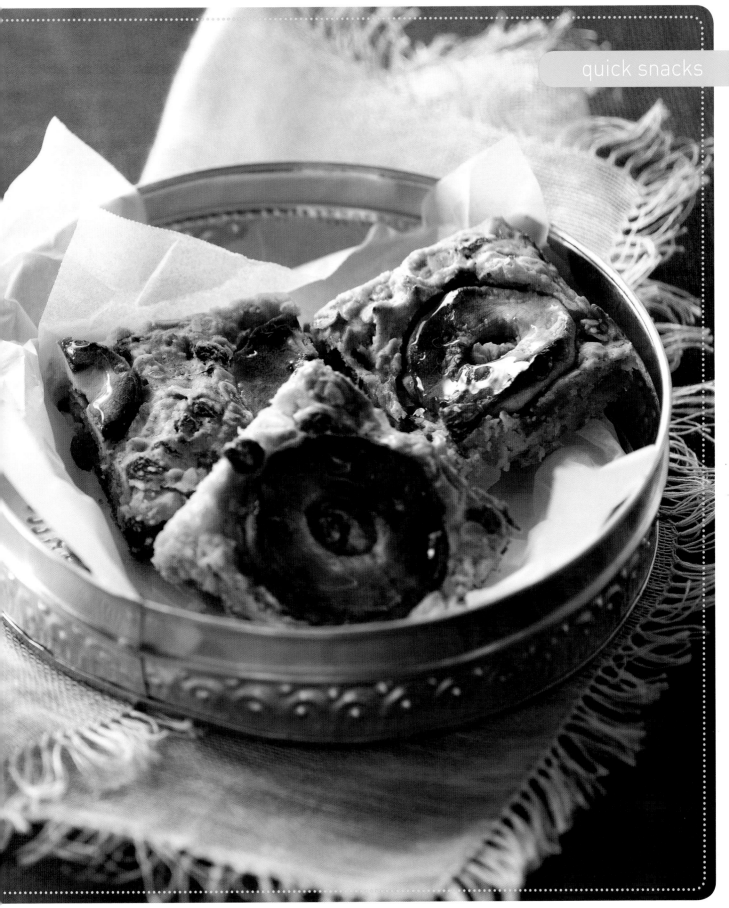

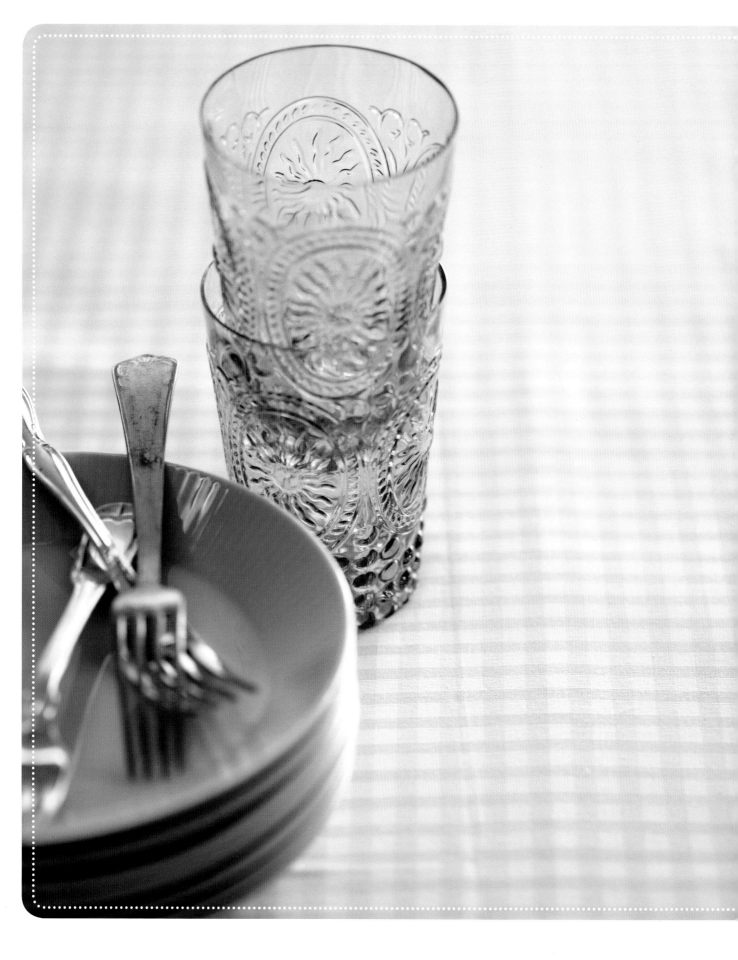

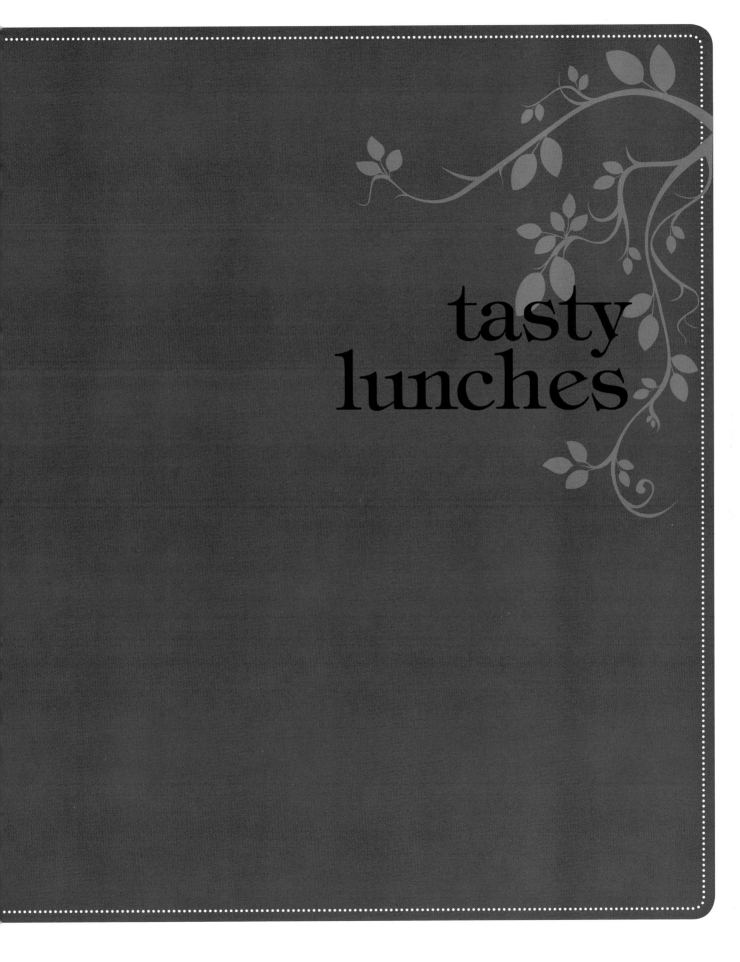

tasty lunches

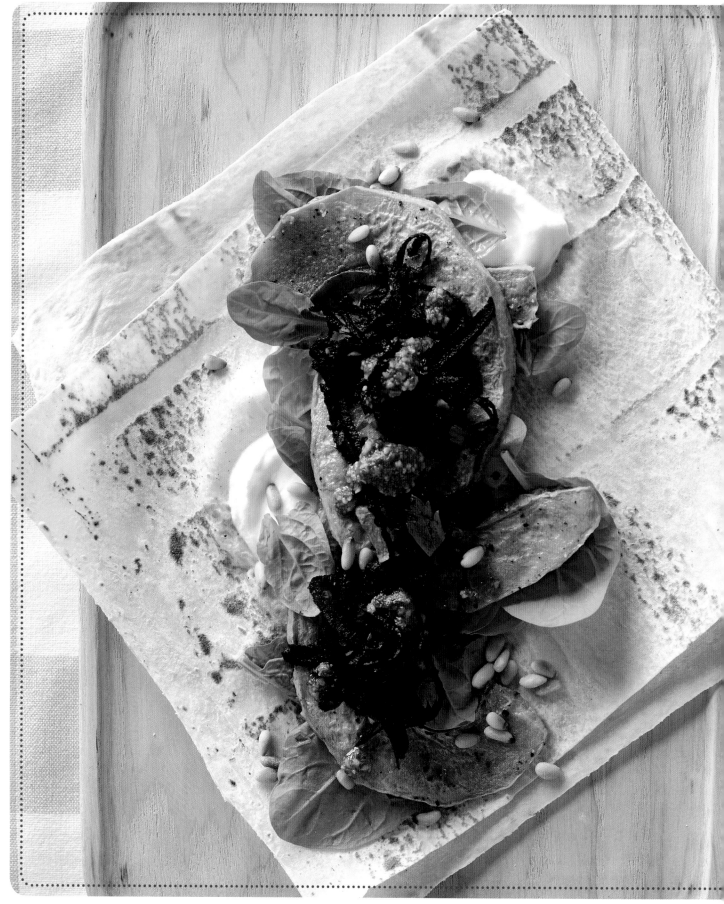

Roasted pumpkin, labne, beetroot and pesto wrap

SERVES 2

200 g pumpkin, peeled and finely sliced

½ tablespoon extra-virgin olive oil

salt and freshly ground black pepper

2 beetroots, peeled and grated

2 tablespoon lemon juice

1 tablespoon flat-leaf parsley, chopped

2 wholemeal pita breads or mountain bread wraps

2 tablespoons labne

50 g baby spinach

2 tablespoons pine nuts, toasted

2 tablespoons pesto

Preheat oven to 180°C.

Place pumpkin slices in a single layer on a lined baking tray. Drizzle with the oil and season with salt and pepper. Roast in the preheated oven for 10–12 minutes, until golden brown and cooked through. Set aside to cool.

Mix the beetroot with the lemon juice and parsley. Season with salt and pepper.

To assemble, lay bread out flat and smear a tablespoon of labne down the middle of each. Cover the bottom three-quarters of the bread with a single layer of pumpkin slices and spread half of the beetroot mix over the pumpkin. Top with spinach leaves, scattered pine nuts and small dollops of pesto. Roll from the filled edge up towards the empty quarter of the bread, taking care to tuck the ingredients in as you go. Cut each roll-up in half and serve.

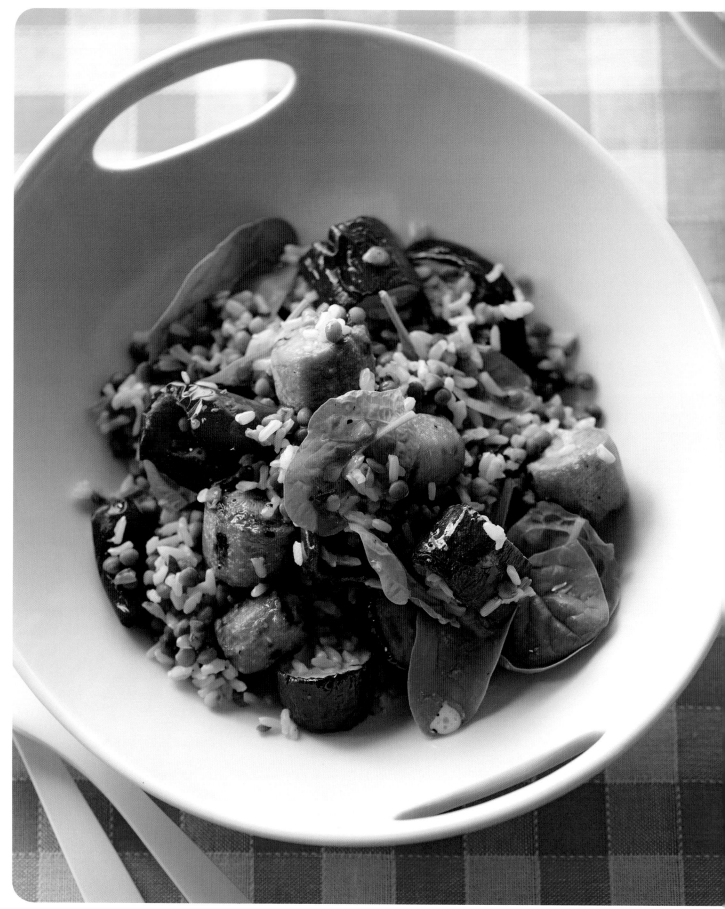

Roasted vegetable, lentil and brown rice salad

SERVES 6

LEMON DRESSING

1 tablespoon lemon juice

½ teaspoon Dijon mustard

60 ml (¼ cup) extra-virgin olive oil

In a bowl, mix the lemon juice and mustard together. Season with salt and freshly ground black pepper, and whisk in the oil.

1 eggplant

salt and freshly ground black pepper

1 red capsicum, deseeded and diced into
  2 cm squares

2 carrots, peeled, halved and thickly sliced

2 zucchini, halved and cut into 2 cm slices

1 red onion, cut into wedges

1 tablespoon of extra-virgin olive oil

100 g (½ cup) brown rice

400 g tin lentils, drained and rinsed

75 g baby spinach

Preheat oven to 180°C.

Cut the eggplants in half and slice to form 1 cm semicircle slices. Sprinkle with salt and set aside until juices bead on the surface, for around 20 minutes. Rinse the eggplant and dry well on paper towels or in a colander.

Toss all the vegetables with the oil, salt and pepper in a baking dish and roast in the preheated oven for 30–40 minutes, or until the vegetables are tender and golden brown. Set aside to cool.

Place the brown rice in a saucepan. Cover with plenty of water and bring to the boil. Reduce to a simmer, cover and cook for 20–30 minutes, or until the rice is tender. Drain and refresh under cold running water.

Mix the vegetables, rice, lentils and spinach leaves together.

Dress and toss just before serving.

Spiced chickpea burgers with fresh beetroot salsa and salad

SERVES 4

BEETROOT SALSA

2 beetroots, peeled and grated

½ tablespoon Dijon mustard

2 tablespoons lemon juice

2 tablespoons fresh chives, chopped

salt and freshly ground black pepper

Combine the mustard and lemon juice in a small bowl and pour over the beetroot. Stir through the chives and season with salt and pepper.

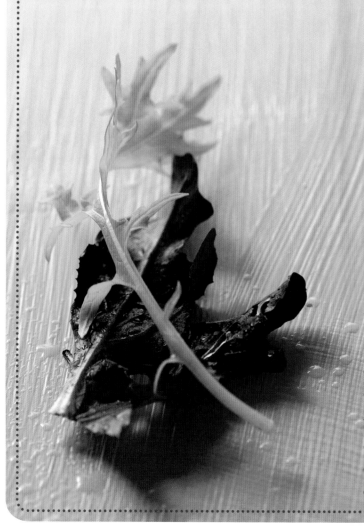

2 tablespoons extra-virgin olive oil

3 onions, sliced

2 teaspoons ground cumin

2 teaspoons ground coriander

1 teaspoon sweet paprika

1 teaspoon chilli powder

100 g baby spinach

400 g tin chickpeas, drained and rinsed

1 egg

½ cup coriander leaves

100–150 g (1–1 ½ cups) breadcrumbs

salt and freshly ground black pepper

4 slices of bread

2 tomatoes, sliced

mixed salad leaves to serve

Heat half of the oil in a large saucepan over a medium heat and add the onion, cumin, coriander, paprika and chilli. Lower the heat and cook for 20 minutes, stirring often, until the onions soften. Add the spinach and cook until wilted.

Combine the spinach, chickpeas, egg, coriander and enough breadcrumbs to bring the mixture together. Season to taste. Divide the mixture into 8 balls and flatten into burger patties.

Heat the remaining oil in a heavy-based frying pan over a medium heat and cook the burgers until golden brown, approximately 5–6 minutes on each side.

To assemble, arrange tomato slices and a handful of salad leaves on each piece of bread. Place two hot chickpea burgers on each piece and top with a spoonful of beetroot salsa.

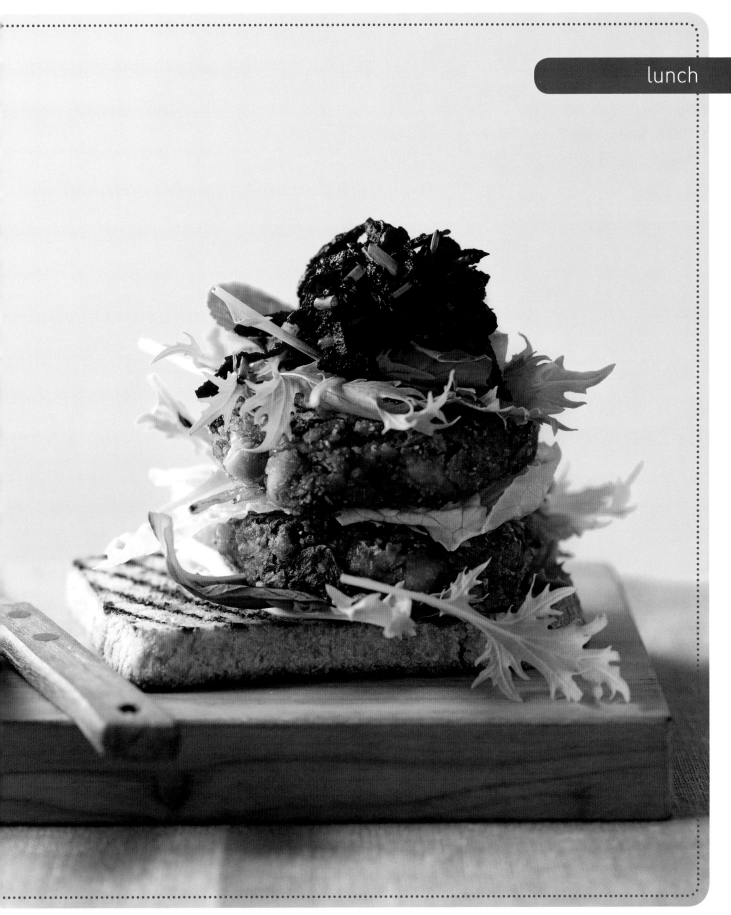

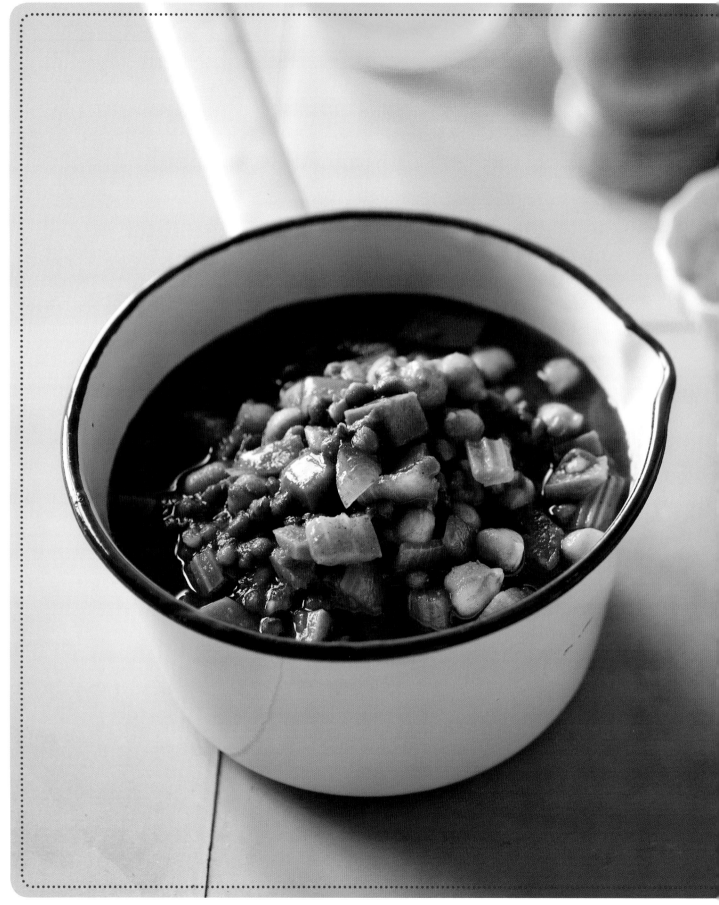

Moroccan chunky chickpea and harissa soup

SERVES 4

1 tablespoon extra-virgin olive oil

1 onion, diced

2 celery stalks, diced into 1 cm pieces

1 carrot, diced into 1 cm cubes

pinch of saffron (optional)

1 teaspoon ground cumin

1 teaspoon ground coriander

1 teaspoon sweet smoked paprika

1 teaspoon harissa

750 ml (3 cups) vegetable or chicken stock

125 ml (½ cup) tomato puree

400 g can chickpeas, drained and rinsed

420 g can lentils, drained and rinsed

¼ cup fresh coriander, chopped

Heat the oil in a large heavy-based saucepan over a medium–high heat. Sauté the onion, celery and carrot until softened, for around 5–6 minutes. Add the spices, harissa and saffron, if using, and cook until fragrant, for around 2–3 minutes. Stir in the stock and tomato puree and bring to the boil. Season, reduce the heat and simmer for 15–20 minutes, stirring often. Add the chickpeas, lentils and coriander and heat through. Check the seasoning and serve hot.

Mexican chicken and bean tortillas with avocado mash

SERVES 4

MARINADE

1 tablespoon extra-virgin olive oil

1 garlic clove, crushed

½ teaspoon salt

½ teaspoon chilli powder

1 teaspoon sweet smoked paprika

½ teaspoon ground coriander

½ teaspoon ground cumin

1 teaspoon mustard powder or mustard seeds, crushed

½ teaspoon freshly ground black pepper

Mix the spices, crushed garlic and oil together. Pour over the chicken and marinate for up to 20 minutes.

CHILLI BEAN SALSA

400 g tin red kidney beans, drained and rinsed

1 small red chilli, deseeded and diced

¼ cup coriander or parsley leaves

½ red onion, finely diced

1 tomato, finely diced

1 tablespoon lime or lemon juice

Mix the beans with the chilli, herbs, onion, tomato and juice together. Set aside.

AVOCADO MASH

1 avocado

2 tablespoons lemon juice

2 tablespoons fresh coriander or flat-leaf parsley, chopped

1 red chilli, deseeded and diced

salt and freshly ground black pepper

Scoop the flesh from the avocado and mash in a bowl with the lemon juice, coriander or parsley, and chilli. Season with salt and freshly ground black pepper, and set aside.

200 g chicken breast fillet, sliced

8 flour tortillas

½ iceberg lettuce, shredded

Heat extra oil in a heavy-based pan over a medium–high heat and sauté the chicken until well browned and cooked through, for around 4–5 minutes.

To assemble, heat the tortillas and place the chicken, chilli beans, lettuce and avocado mash on the bottom third. Fold the tortilla sides inwards to meet in the middle, then roll up from the bottom. Slice diagonally through the middle and serve.

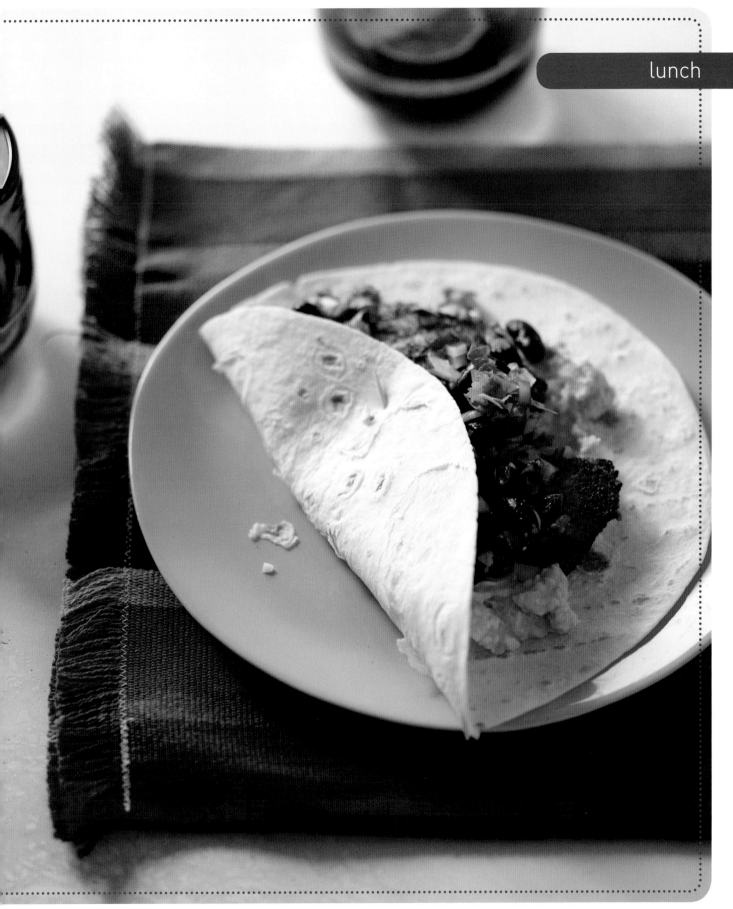

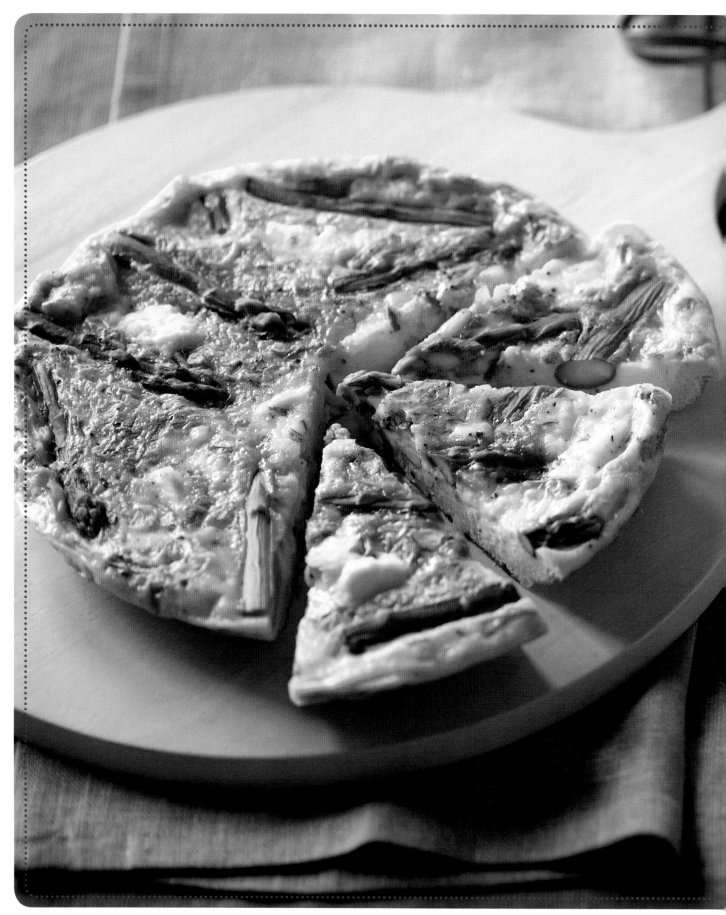

Asparagus and ricotta frittata

SERVES 4

2 tablespoons extra-virgin olive oil

1 onion, finely diced

6 eggs

25 g (¼ cup) parmesan, grated

2 tablespoons flat-leaf parsley, chopped

200 g asparagus, trimmed and cut into 5 cm lengths

50 g ricotta

Preheat oven to 180°C.

Heat the oil in a small, ovenproof frying pan over a medium heat. Sauté the onion until slightly softened. Allow to cool.

Beat together eggs, parmesan, herbs and onion. Pour into the frying pan, scatter asparagus over the top and add spoonfuls of ricotta. Cook on the stovetop until the base sets, for around 4–5 minutes. Place the pan in the preheated oven to finish cooking the top, for about 10–15 minutes.

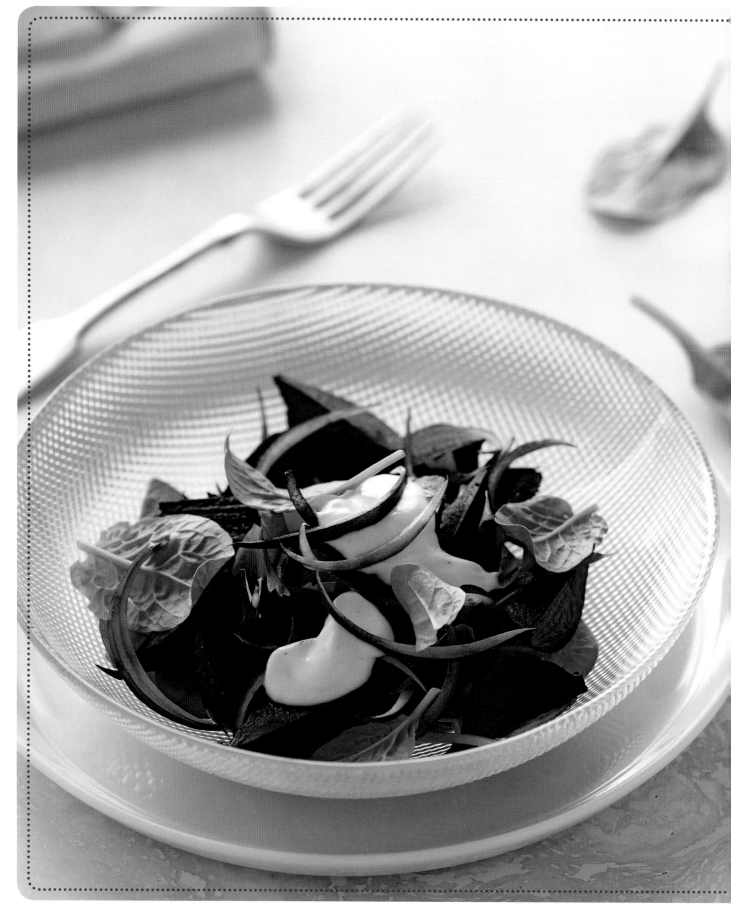

Beetroot, spinach and yoghurt salad

SERVES 2

YOGHURT DRESSING

180 g (¾ cup) natural yoghurt

2 tablespoon lemon juice

2 garlic cloves, crushed

1 tablespoon tahini

salt and freshly ground black pepper

Mix all the ingredients together. Keep refrigerated.

3 beetroots, leaves trimmed

100 g baby spinach

½ red onion, finely sliced

Place the beetroots in a saucepan, cover with water and bring to the boil. Reduce the heat, cover with a lid and cook for 30–40 minutes, until tender. Drain, allow to cool, then peel and cut into wedges.

Place the spinach in a bowl and add the beetroot wedges and onion slices. Drizzle the yoghurt dressing over to serve.

delicious
dinners

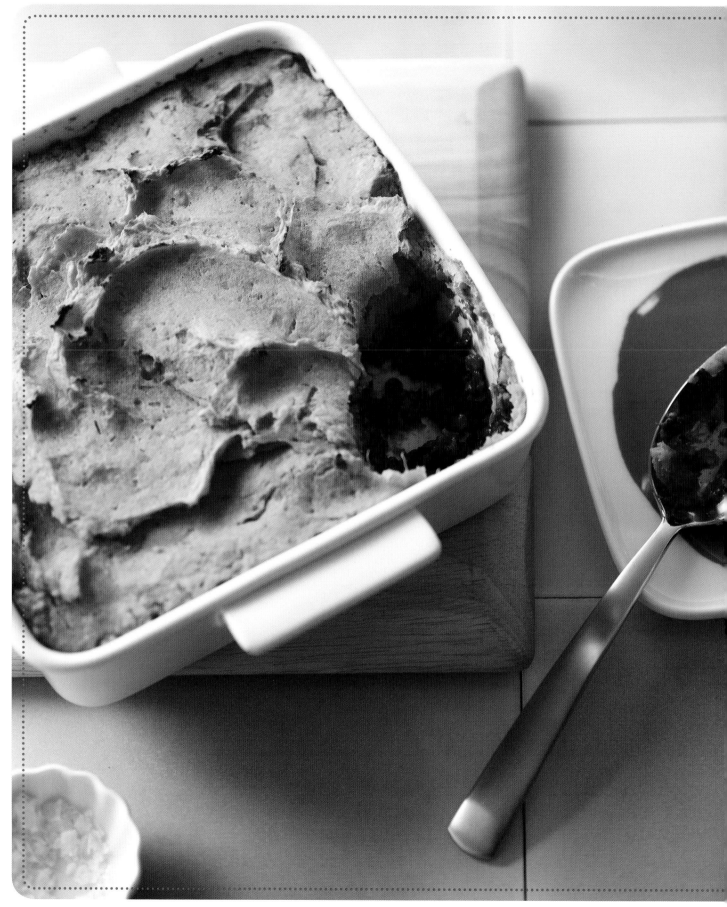

Moroccan lentil and sweet potato shepherd's pie

SERVES 4

½ tablespoon extra-virgin olive oil

1 onion, diced

1 garlic clove, crushed

2 teaspoons harissa

1 teaspoon ground coriander

1 teaspoon ground cumin

250 g (1 cup) French-style green lentils

750 ml (3 cups) vegetable stock

125 ml (½ cup) tomato puree

salt and freshly ground black pepper

¼ cup chopped coriander leaves

600 g sweet potatoes, peeled and diced

Heat oil in a medium-sized saucepan over a medium–high heat and sauté the onion for 3–4 minutes. Add the garlic, harissa, coriander and cumin, and cook for a further 1–2 minutes, stirring often. Add the lentils, stock and tomato puree, and bring to the boil. Reduce the heat and simmer for 45 minutes, stirring occasionally, until the lentils are cooked and the sauce is reduced. Season to taste and stir through the coriander leaves at the end.

Preheat oven to 180ºC.

To prepare the topping, simmer the sweet potatoes in a saucepan of water until tender, for about 10 minutes. Drain and mash, then season with salt and pepper.

Pour the lentil mixture into a 2-litre, deep baking dish. Cover with the mashed sweet potato and bake in the preheated oven for 20 minutes, or until crispy and golden brown on top.

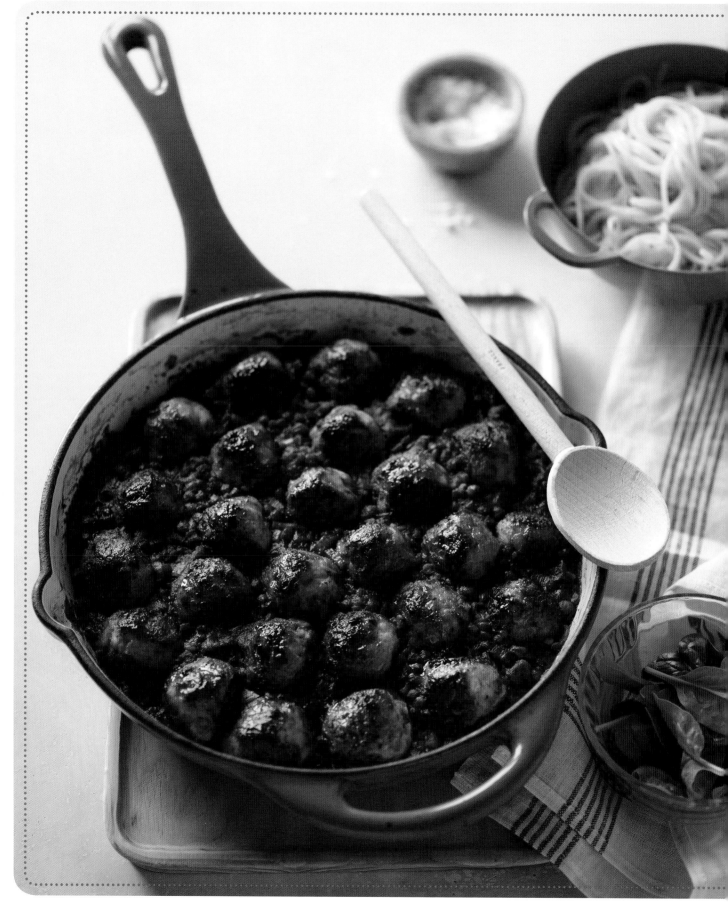

Braised meatballs with lentils and spinach

SERVES 4

500 g chicken mince

100 g (½ cup) ricotta

¼ teaspoon freshly grated nutmeg

1 egg

50 g (½ cup) breadcrumbs

salt and freshly ground black pepper

1 tablespoon extra-virgin olive oil

1 onion, diced

1 garlic clove, crushed

250 ml (1 cup) chicken stock

250 ml (1 cup) tomato puree

400 g tin lentils, drained and rinsed

100 g baby spinach

2 tablespoons flat-leaf parsley, chopped

spaghetti to serve

Preheat oven to 180°C.

Mix chicken mince, ricotta, nutmeg, egg and breadcrumbs in a bowl. Season with salt and freshly ground black pepper. Combine well and roll into small meatballs.

Heat half a tablespoon of the oil in a heavy-based frying pan over a medium heat and sauté meatballs, turning often, until golden brown, for 5–6 minutes. Transfer meatballs to a deep baking dish.

Return the pan to the heat (it doesn't have to be clean), add the remaining oil and diced onion, and cook until soft. Add the garlic, stock and tomato puree, and bring to the boil. Stir in the lentils and pour mixture over the meatballs. Cover with foil and bake in the preheated oven for 30 minutes.

To serve, stir through the spinach and parsley, check the seasoning, and ladle over hot spaghetti.

Seared swordfish with avocado salsa

SERVES 4

AVOCADO SALSA

1 avocado, peeled, and diced

2 tablespoons coriander leaves

2 tablespoons lime juice

2 spring onions, finely sliced

1 tomato, finely diced

1 dash Tabasco sauce (optional)

salt and freshly ground black pepper

Place all the ingredients in a bowl and stir very gently to combine.

4 swordfish steaks

1 tablespoon extra-virgin olive oil

salt and freshly ground black pepper

wild rocket or baby spinach to serve

lime wedges to serve

Heat a chargrill or frying pan over a high heat. Season the fish with the oil, salt and pepper and grill until just cooked through, for 2–3 minutes each side. Serve with the avocado salsa, green leaves and lime wedges.

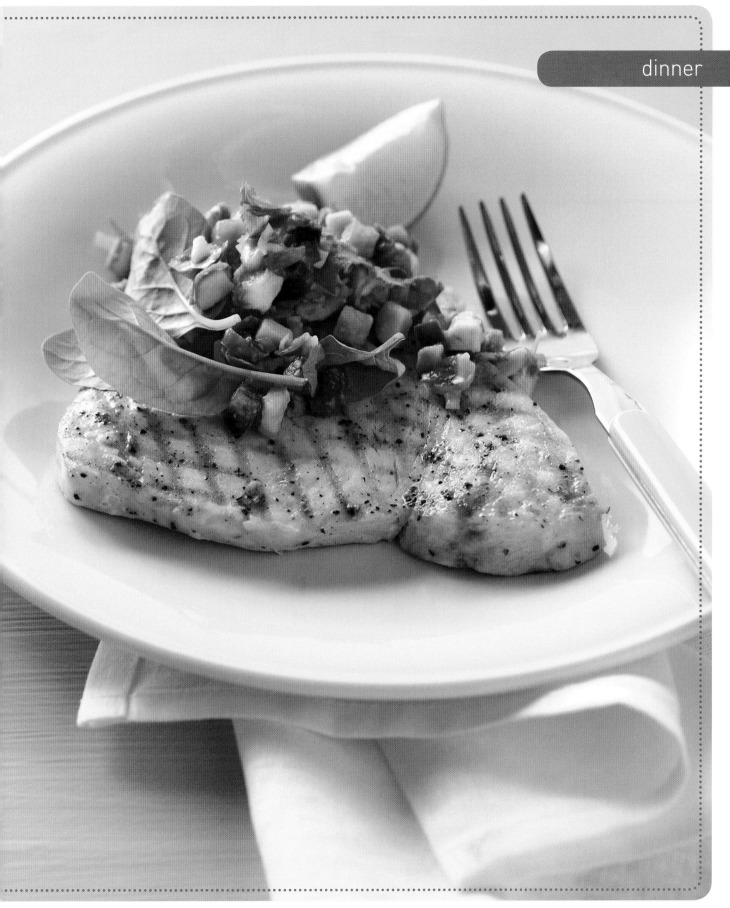

Asian vegetable and soba noodle salad

SERVES 4

ASIAN DRESSING
zest of 2 limes, grated
60 ml (¼ cup) lime juice
60 ml (¼ cup) rice wine vinegar
60 ml (¼ cup) fish sauce
80 ml (⅓ cup) sweet chilli sauce

Mix the lime zest, juice, vinegar and fish sauce. Add the sweet chilli sauce and stir to combine. Store in the refrigerator until needed.

270 g soba noodles
1 bunch broccolini
100 g snow peas
1 carrot, peeled into long shavings
½ red capsicum, finely sliced
¼ red cabbage, finely sliced
1 cup bean sprouts
⅓ cup coriander leaves
¼ cup mint leaves (regular or Vietnamese)
4 spring onions, finely sliced

To prepare the salad, bring a pot of water to the boil, add soba noodles and cook until tender, for about 4 minutes. Drain and refresh under cold running water.

Bring another pot of water to the boil, add the broccolini and cook for 1 minute. Add the snow peas and boil for a further 1–2 minutes. Drain and refresh.

Slice broccolini and snow peas into long lengths and add to the noodles along with the carrot, capsicum, cabbage, bean sprouts, herbs and spring onions. Pour over enough dressing to coat, toss to combine, and serve.

You can add 200 g marinated tofu to the salad for extra protein.

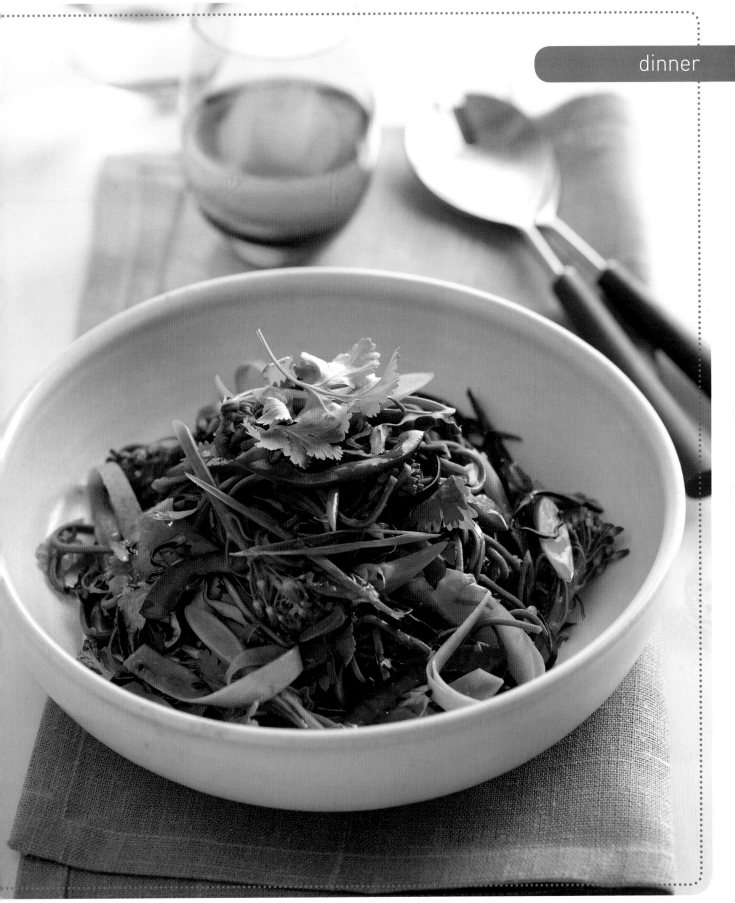

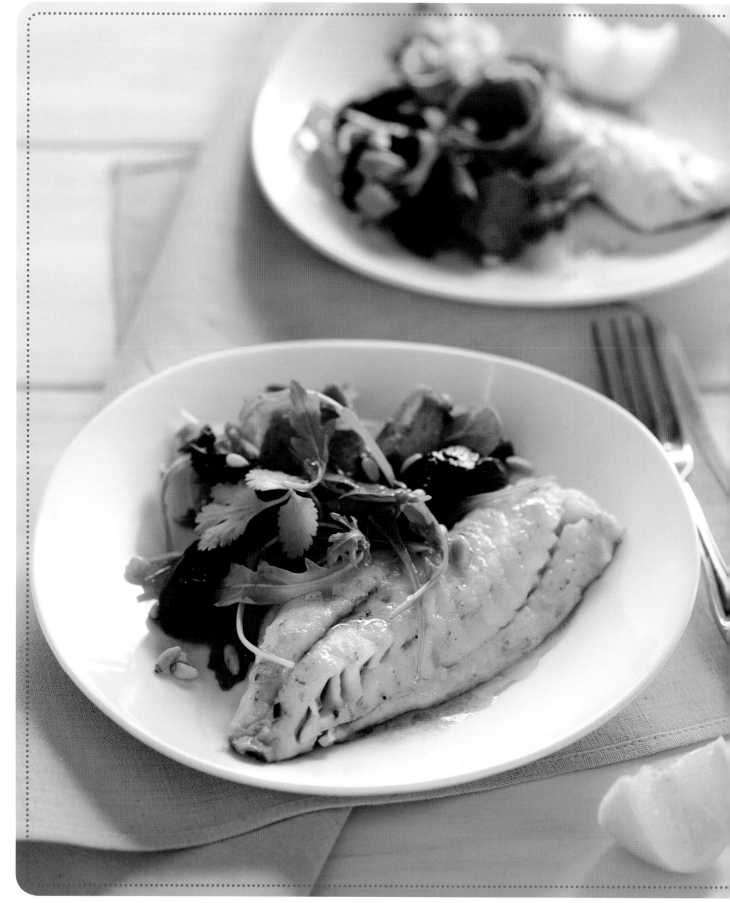

Snapper with spinach and pumpkin salad

SERVES 4

200 g pumpkin, peeled and diced into 2 cm pieces

1 tablespoon extra-virgin olive oil

salt and freshly ground black pepper

1 red capsicum

75 g baby spinach

75 g wild rocket

⅓ cup coriander leaves

⅓ cup flat-leaf parsley leaves

75 g (½ cup) pine nuts, toasted

½ preserved lemon, soaked and pulp removed, finely diced, optional

4 × 150 g snapper fillets

pomegranate dressing (page 154)

salt and freshly ground black pepper

Preheat oven to 180°C.

Lay pumpkin on a baking tray, drizzle with half the oil, and season with salt and freshly ground black pepper. Roast in the preheated oven for 20–25 minutes, until tender. Set aside to cool slightly.

Place capsicum on a baking tray, brush with the remaining oil and roast in the preheated oven, turning once or twice, until skin blisters, for about 20 minutes. Place the capsicum in a plastic bag to steam the skin. When cool, slip skin away and remove the seeds. Slice flesh into ½ cm thick slices.

Combine the pumpkin, capsicum, spinach, rocket, herbs, pine nuts and preserved lemon, if using, in a large bowl.

Heat extra oil in a heavy-based frying pan over a medium–high heat and sauté fish fillets until golden brown and cooked through, for 3–4 minutes on each side. Season with salt and freshly ground black pepper.

To serve, pour over enough dressing to coat the salad and toss to combine. Divide the salad and fish between four plates, and serve with a wedge of lemon each.

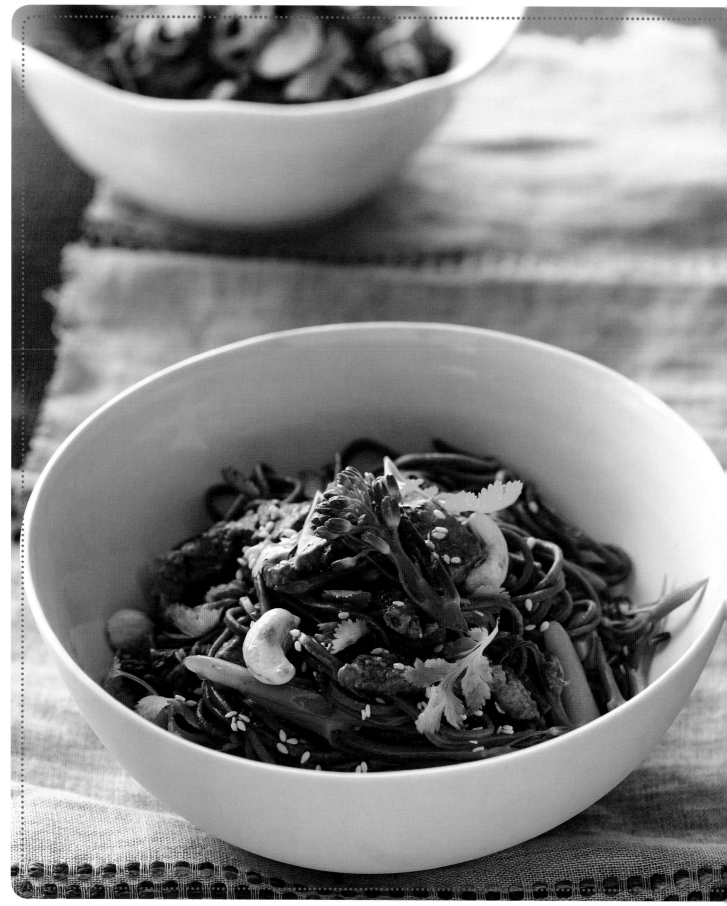

Stir-fried ginger beef with broccolini and cashews

SERVES 2

2 tablespoons soy sauce

1 tablespoon sesame oil

1 tablespoon grated ginger

200 g beef fillet, cut into strips

½ tablespoon extra-virgin olive oil

180 g soba noodles

2 spring onions, finely sliced

1 bunch broccolini, cut into 2 cm chunks

75 g (½ cup) cashew nuts, toasted

¼ cup coriander leaves

1 teaspoon sesame seeds, toasted

Whisk together soy sauce, sesame oil and ginger. Pour half over the beef strips and leave to marinate for up to 20 minutes. Keep remaining half aside.

Bring a pot of water to the boil and cook the noodles for 3–4 minutes, until al dente. Drain and mix with the reserved marinade.

While the noodles are cooking, heat the oil in a wok over a high heat and sauté the spring onions briefly. Add the beef strips and stir-fry until browned all over, for 3–4 minutes. Add the broccolini and cashew nuts, cover with a lid and cook for a further 2 minutes. Add the cooked noodles, coriander and sesame seeds, and toss to combine.

Chilli and soy stir-fried kangaroo with bok choy

SERVES 4

1 × 450 g kangaroo sirloin

1 tablespoon peanut oil

250 g bok choy

80 ml (⅓ cup) sweet chilli sauce

80 ml (⅓ cup) light soy sauce

3 spring onions, green top only, finely sliced

steamed rice to serve

Divide sirloin down the centre into two pieces. Trim any white sinew and slice on an angle into 1 cm slices.

Heat the peanut oil in a wok over a high heat. Add the kangaroo and stir-fry for 1 minute. Add the bok choy, chilli sauce, soy sauce and spring onion. Stir well and allow to heat through. Serve with steamed rice.

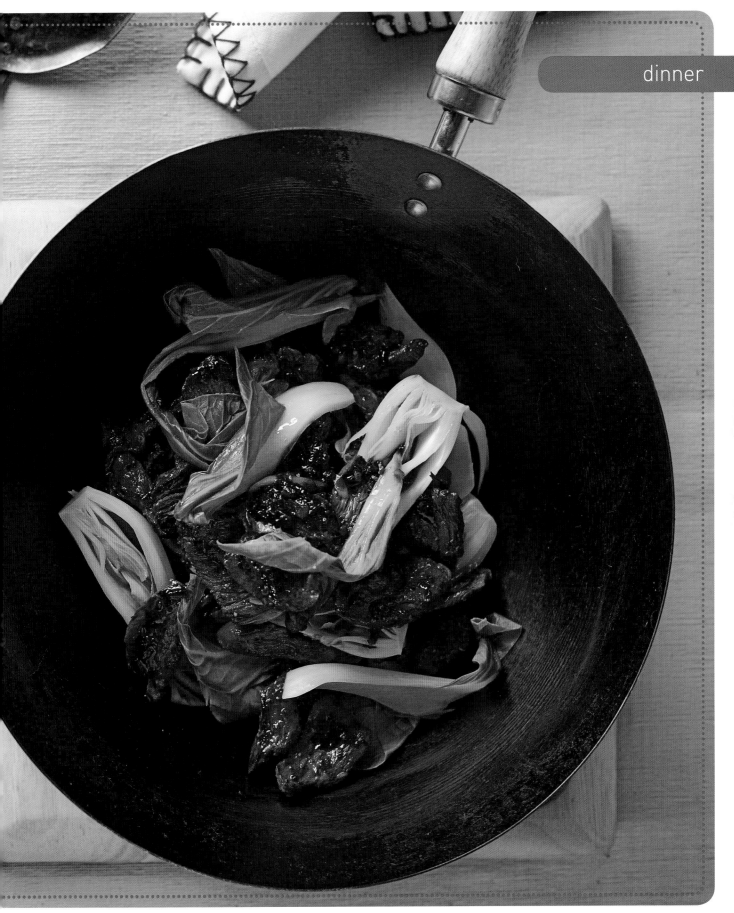

Spiced sweet potato and chickpea patties with yoghurt dressing

MAKES 8

500 g sweet potato, peeled and diced

salt and freshly ground black pepper

4 spring onions, finely sliced

1 teaspoon ground cumin

1 teaspoon ground coriander

1 teaspoon sweet smoked paprika

1 egg, lightly beaten

1 cup wholemeal breadcrumbs

2 tablespoons flat-leaf parsley, chopped

400 g tin chickpeas, drained and rinsed

2 tablespoons plain flour

3 teaspoons sesame seeds

½ tablespoon extra-virgin olive oil

lemon wedges to serve

broccolini to serve

yoghurt dressing (page 177)

Simmer the sweet potatoes in a saucepan of water until tender, for about 10 minutes. Drain and mash. Season with salt and pepper.

Mix the spring onions, spices, egg, breadcrumbs, parsley and chickpeas into the mashed sweet potato. Divide the mixture into eight equal portions and shape into patties approximately 1.5 cm thick.

Combine the flour and sesame seeds on a plate. Roll the patties in the flour mixture, shaking off any excess. Heat the oil in a large frying pan over medium heat. Sauté the patties, in batches if necessary, for 3–4 minutes on each side until golden brown. Place in a preheated oven to keep warm.

Serve the patties with yoghurt dressing, lemon wedges and steamed broccolini.

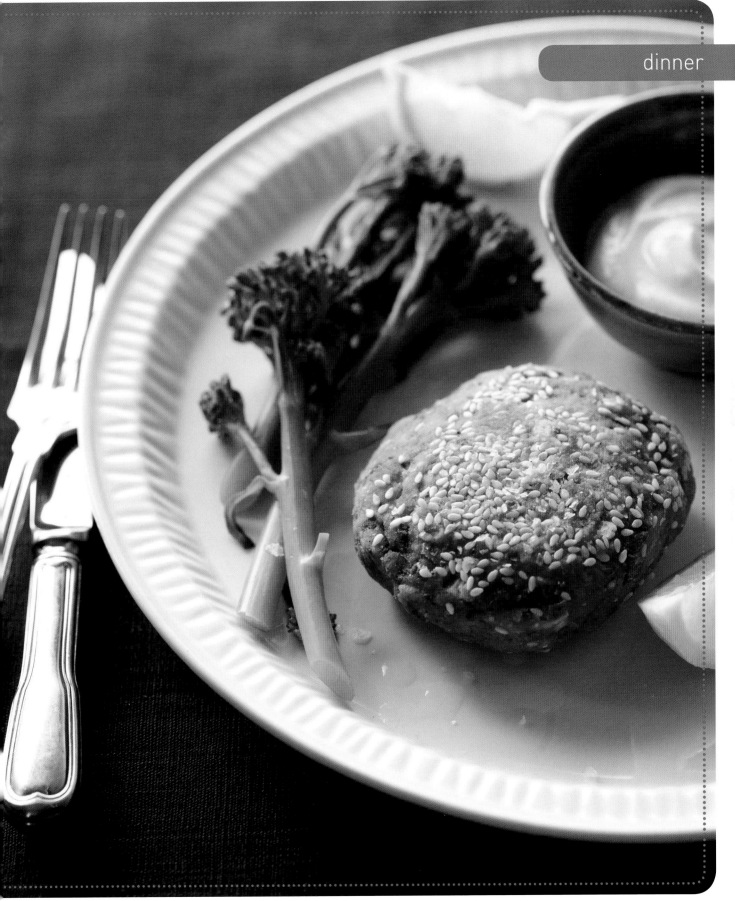

Fish parcels with lemongrass, coriander, chilli and Asian greens

SERVES 4

250 g bok choy, sliced into long strips

½ red capsicum, finely sliced

1 carrot, julienned

2 tablespoons soy sauce

½ teaspoon sesame oil

1 teaspoon grated ginger

1 lemongrass stem, white part only,
  finely sliced

2 red chillies, finely diced

4 × 150 g firm white fish fillets
  (such as blue eye or snapper)

4 greaseproof paper squares

12–16 coriander sprigs

steamed jasmine rice to serve

Preheat oven to 180°C.

Combine the bok choy, capsicum and carrot.

Mix together the soy sauce, sesame oil, ginger, lemongrass and chillies. Brush the mixture over the fish fillets.

Lay the four greaseproof paper squares out flat. Divide most of the vegetables between them, making a pile in the middle of each sheet.

Rest one piece of fish on top of each pile of vegetables and top with remaining vegetables and 3 or 4 sprigs of coriander. Fold two paper ends in to the middle and pull remaining two edges up together. Roll paper ends over tightly to secure on top of the parcels. Bake in the preheated oven for 15 minutes.

Serve with jasmine rice.

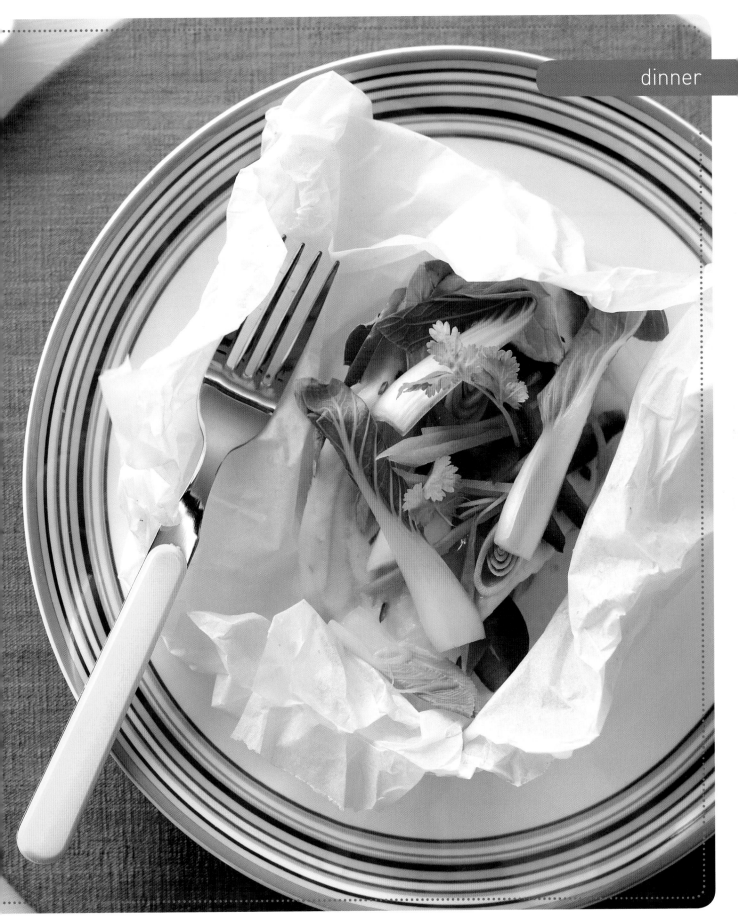

Index

acetate 37
acne 111
addiction
   sugar 31, 51
adenosine tri-phosphate 63
adrenal glands 77
adrenaline 55
aerobic 63, 66
alcohol 37, 47, 57, 58, 77, 94, 127
alkaline 18
allicin 57
amino acids 22, 35
anaerobic 63, 66
antibodies 55
appetite 51, 52, 54, 58
apple 88
artifical
   colours 86, 101
   flavours 86, 101
   sweeteners 32, 35, 36, 86, 101
     mannitol 36, 101
     aspartame 35, 36, 101
avocado 30

binge eating 24, 29, 83
blood sugar 26, 32, 33, 50, 51, 54, 67, 77, 86
blood pressure 30, 43, 55
bread 23, 47
breakfast 33, 47, 57, 92, 95, 102

caffeine 38, 45, 57, 60
cake 84
canola oil 29, 30
carbohydrate 22, 26, 29, 31, 33, 37, 43, 55, 57, 77, 102
carbon monoxide 55
cardiovascular 66
cereal 88
chocolate 47, 55, 84, 85
cholesterol 23, 24, 29, 30
cilia 55
coffee 38, 43, 45, 60
condiments 43, 118
copper 47
corn syrup 35
cravings 103, 104

crying 55
dehydration 40, 45, 60
depression 14, 29, 55
dextrose 36
diabetes 26, 33, 36, 51, 56, 58
diuretic 43, 44, 60
dopamine 55

eat naked 18, 118, 119, 126
eating disorders 29
electrolytes 45
emotional eating 14, 24, 86, 89, 103
energy 10, 22, 29, 63
energy bars 94
energy drinks 43, 45
exercise 22, 58, 63, 66, 67, 69, 70, 72, 76, 77, 79, 86, 114, 125

fad diets 18, 21, 22, 29
family 106, 107, 109
fast food 30, 43, 47, 124,125
fat 22, 26, 29–33, 43, 70, 72, 102
  burn 29, 32, 50, 52, 54, 58, 66, 67, 76, 125
  cells 29, 32, 51, 52
  fat-free 31, 32, 82, 102
  low-fat 26, 57, 102
  visceral 29
fats
  good 24, 26, 29
  healthy 47
  mono-unsaturated 24, 26, 29, 30
  omega-3 24, 30
  omega-6 30
  polyunsaturated 26, 30
  trans 30, 36
  unsaturated 30
fatty acids 29, 30, 32, 33, 43, 51
fatty liver disease 33
fibre 102
fish 21
  oil 29
fitness 79
  coach 79
  journal 79
  test 73
flaxseeds 23, 29, 30, 57, 88
free-range 21
fructose 26, 31–33, 36, 43, 57, 100

glucose   22, 31, 32, 33, 43, 51, 63, 67, 104
glucuronoactone   45
gluten   57
glycaemic index (GI)   23, 26
glycogen   22, 56, 58
goals   11, 12, 79
grapefruit   88
green tea   88, 95

habits   12, 42, 84, 91, 94, 111, 119, 122
heart-rate monitor   74
High fructose corn syrup (HFCS)   35
hormones   22, 24, 26, 29, 31, 32, 40, 50, 51, 52, 54–58, 60, 67, 79, 100
    anabolic   54
    cholecystokinin (CKK)   31, 32
    cortisol   32, 37, 54–57, 63
    endogenous opioids   103
    endorphins   9, 55, 58, 63, 79
    epinephrine   54
    ghrelin   33, 50–52, 57, 58
    human growth (HGH)   52, 58, 63
    imbalance   56
    leptin   32, 33, 50, 51, 57, 58
    lycopene   47
    melatonin   77
    norepinephrine   54
    oestrogen   54, 57
    oestrone   54
    oxytocin   55
    serotonin   55, 77, 104, 125
    testosterone   37, 54, 57, 63
hydrogenation   30, 36, 101
hypoglycaemia   77

immune system   32, 45, 52, 55
insulin   26, 32, 33, 43, 50, 51, 54, 60, 63

journal   11, 14, 79, 83, 88
juice   36, 43, 47
junk food   18, 103

kissing   55

lactose   33
labels   36, 100, 102
laughing   55

licorice   57
libido   92
meditation   117, 118
metabolism   21, 24, 31, 33, 43, 50, 54, 57, 58, 60, 63, 67, 70
metabolic syndrome   32, 56, 58
motivation   83
muscle   21, 52, 54, 63, 69, 70, 72

niacin   57
nitrates   21, 100, 101
nude food   18, 47, 50, 95
nutrients
    water-soluble   47
nuts   24, 29, 30, 35, 43, 47, 57, 94

obesity   32
oil
    olive   29, 30
    safflower   30
    sesame   30
    soybean   30
omega-3   21, 57, 88
oxytocin   55

pancreas   51
phosphate   38
portion sizes   24, 25, 92, 96
Premenstrual Dysphoric Disorder (PMDD)   56
Premenstrual Syndrome (PMS)   56
preservatives   100, 101
protein   21, 22, 24, 29, 30–32, 43, 57, 67, 95, 97, 102

relaxation   10
restaurants   91, 127
resting pose   124

saccharin   35, 36, 101
salt   32, 43, 100, 101, 103
scales   69
shortening   36
sleep   24, 37, 52, 58, 86
smoking   55, 58,
soba noodles   47
sodium   43, 103, 104
soft drinks   36, 38, 43, 47, 127
soup   45, 111

spices   35
sports drinks   45
starvation response   21, 22, 95
stress   54, 56, 60, 86, 117, 119, 122
stretches   117, 120–122
sucralose   35, 36
sucrose   33, 36, 43
sugar   26, 30–32, 35, 36, 43, 67, 88, 102
sweat   67
sweet cravings   24, 35, 104

taekwondo   4
tar   55
taurine   45
3–2–1 rule   24
thyroid   50, 51, 56, 63,
triglycerides   33
time   14
thermoregulation   77
tomatoes   47
training   9, 66, 69,
    abdominal   72
    cardio   66, 67, 75, 77
    circuit   66, 69, 92
    cross   77
    interval   66, 73, 77
    resistance   70, 74
    strength   75, 77
    weight   72, 77
type-2 diabetes   33

vegetables   45, 57, 94
vitamins   29, 57
visualisation   10

water   24, 36, 40, 43, 45, 47, 89, 95
warrior
    weapons   3
    code   4
    cry   10
    pose   120, 122
    scrolls   11
    spirit   8
weights   69, 72
white flour   23
wholegrains   23

zinc   57

Index to Recipes

Almond and apricot muesli   145
almonds   133, 145
Asian vegetable and soba noodle salad   186
Asparagus and ricotta frittata   175
asparagus   133, 175
Avocado and roasted tomato on toast   139
avocado   139, 172, 184
beans   172
beef   191
beetroot   165, 168, 177
Beetroot, spinach and yoghurt salad   177
blueberries   134, 140
bok choy   192
Braised meatballs with lentils and spinach   183
Breakfast quinoa with summer fruits   143
broccolini   191
burgers   168
burghul   154

capsicum   136
carrots   158
chicken   172, 183
chickpeas   154, 158, 168, 171, 194
chilli   172, 192, 196
Chilli and soy stir-fried kangaroo with bok choy   192
Cinnamon porridge with blueberries and honey   140

dried fruit   145, 150, 152, 160
dressing
    Asian   186
    pomegranate   154
yoghurt   194
dukkah   133

Eggwhite omelette with spinach, capsicum
    and mushroom   136
eggs
    eggwhite omlette   136
    soft boiled   133

Fig and almond balls   150
fish   196
    snapper   189
    swordfish   184
Fish parcels with lemongrass, coriander, chilli and asian
    greens   196
frittata   175
fruit   143
    pomegranate   154
    strawberries   149

Fruity oat slice   160

Hearty tabbouleh   154
hummus   158

kangaroo   192

labne   165
lentils   167, 181, 183

marinade   172
meatballs   183
Mexican chicken and bean tortillas with avocado
    mash   172
Moroccan chunky chickpea and harissa soup   171
Moroccan lentil and sweet potato shepherd's pie   181
muesli   145
Muesli slice   152
muffins   157
mushrooms   136

pancakes   134
patties   194
pesto   165
porridge   140
pumpkin   157, 165, 189
Pumpkin, cardamom and cashew muffins   157

quinoa   143

rice, brown   167
Roasted carrot hummus with fresh tomato salsa   158
Roasted pumpkin, labne, beetroot and pesto wrap   165
Roasted vegetable, lentil and brown rice salad   167

salad   168
    roasted vegetable, lentil and brown rice   167
    spinach and pumpkin salad   189
salsa
    avocado   184
    beetroot   168
    chilli bean   172
    tomato   158
Seared swordfish with avocado salsa   184
shepherd's pie   181
slices
    fruity oat   160
muesli   152
Snapper with spinach and pumpkin salad   189
soba noodles   186, 191
Soft boiled eggs with grilled asparagus and dukkah   133
soup   171
Spiced chickpea burgers with fresh beetroot salsa and
Spiced sweet potato and chickpea patties with yoghurt
    dressing   194
spinach   136, 177, 183, 189
Stir-fried ginger beef with broccolini and cashews   191
strawberries   143, 149
Strawberries with balsamic vinegar   149
sweet potato   181, 194

tabbouleh   154
toast   139
tomato   139
tortillas   172

vegetables
    Asian   186, 196
roasted   167

Wholewheat blueberry pancakes   134
wrap   165

Dedicated to my warrior tribe: Dad, my true Warrior Chief who taught me everything I know. Mum, my Warrior Goddess who taught me that real strength is gentle. To my beautiful sister Bridget and little bro Lleyton—fight for what you love and be yourselves out there. To my darling Edward Kavalee, who reminds me that as a warrior the only arms I need are for hugging. Love you all. Much!

Warrior thanks to the team at Hardie Grant for their samurai speed, precision and heart. My agent Clare Forster at Curtis Brown, for getting her ninja on to do this project. My forever friend Emily Royal who is always by my side in any battle; thank you for your loving edits. My dear friend Elena Jacovides who inspires me to attempt Kitchen Kung Fu. Thanks to our Ninja Army—the students at Hall's Taekwondo, far and wide, who are unleashing their inner warriors and earning their black belts in health.

Go ninjas, go ninjas, go!

Tiffiny